NCLEX-RN®: Medications You Need to Know for the Exam

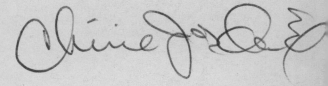

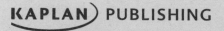

KAPLAN) PUBLISHING

New York

Related Kaplan Books for Nurses

NCLEX-RN®: Strategies for the Registered Nursing Licensing Exam, 2008–2009 Edition
Your Career in Nursing
First Year Nurse

NCLEX-RN®: Medications You Need to Know for the Exam

Barbara Arnoldussen, R.N., M.B.A.

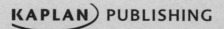

KAPLAN PUBLISHING

New York

© 2008 Kaplan, Inc.

Published by Kaplan Publishing, a division of Kaplan, Inc.
1 Liberty Plaza, 24th Floor
New York, NY 10006

Printed in the United States of America

June 2008
10 9 8 7 6 5

ISBN-13: 978-1-4277-9747-6

Kaplan Publishing books are available at special quantity discounts to use for sales promotions, employee premiums, or educational purposes. Please email our Special Sales Department to order or for more information at kaplanpublishing@kaplan.com, or write to Kaplan Publishing, 1 Liberty Plaza, 24th Floor, New York, NY 10006.

Table of Contents

The following categories have been included in the book, listed in alphabetical order by category.

HOW TO USE THIS BOOK

Kaplan NCLEX-RN®: Medications You Need to Know for the Exam is perfectly designed to help you learn important information about 296 essential medications in a quick, easy, and fun way. Simply read the medication's category, subcategory, generic and brand names, and the phonetic pronunciation of the generic name on the front of each page; then flip to the back to see its side effects, usage, and other important nursing considerations.

Disclaimer

The material in this book is intended for study and test preparation purposes only. This book is under no circumstances to be used to prescribe medication, provide medical treatment and/or therapy, or treat patients or any other individuals in any way. The publisher is not responsible for use of this book in any manner other than its intended purpose as a study guide.

CETIRIZINE HCL
(seh-<u>teer</u>-uh-zene)
(Zyrtec)

• •

FEXOFENADINE
(fex-oh-<u>fi</u>-na-deen)
(Allegra)

Side Effects
  Drowsiness
  Fatigue
  Dry mouth

Nursing Considerations
  Relief of seasonal allergic
  rhinitis symptoms
  Relief of perennial allergic
  rhinitis caused by molds,
  animal dander, and other
  allergens
  Avoid alcohol during
  cetirizine therapy
  Rx; Preg Cat B

• •

Side Effects
  Drowsiness

Nursing Considerations
  Management of rhinitis,
  allergy symptoms, chronic
  idiopathic urticaria
  Avoid alcohol, other CNS
  depressants
  60 mg tablet: onset within
  1 hour, peak 2–3 hours,
  duration about 12 hours
  180 mg tablet: duration
  24 hours
  Rx; Preg Cat C

HYDROXYZINE
(hye-<u>drox</u>-i-zeen)
(Atarax, Vistaril)

• •

LORATADINE
(lor-<u>a</u>-ti-deen)
(Claritin)

Side Effects
  Drowsiness, dry mouth

Nursing Considerations
  Treatment of pruritus,
  pre-op anxiety, post-op
  nausea and vomiting, to
  potentiate opioid analgesics,
  sedation
  PO: onset 15–30 minutes,
  duration 4–6 hours
  Avoid use with alcohol,
  other CNS depressants
  Teach pt. dizziness/drowsi-
  ness may occur; use caution
  in potentially hazardous
  activities
  Rx; Preg Cat C

• •

Side Effects
  Drowsiness

Nursing Considerations
  Management of seasonal
  rhinitis
  Avoid alcohol, other CNS
  depressants
  Take on empty stomach
  1 hour before or 2 hours
  after meals
  Onset 1–3 hours, peak
  8–12 hours, duration greater
  than or equal to 24 hours
  Rx/OTC; Preg Cat B

BECLOMETHASONE
(be-kloe-<u>meth</u>-a-sone)
(Beclovent, Beconase)

• •

FLUNISOLIDE
(floo-<u>niss</u>-oh-lide)
(Nasolide, Aerobid)

Side Effects
Dystonia, hoarseness
Oropharyngeal fungal
infections
Headache
Sore throat
Dyspepsia

Nursing Considerations
Used in chronic asthma
treatment, seasonal or
perennial rhinitis
Nasal spray: onset 5–7 days,
(up to 3 weeks in some
patients), peak up to 3
weeks
Inhaler: onset 10 minutes
Use regular peak flow
monitoring to determine
respiratory status
Rx; Preg Cat C

• •

Side Effects
Dysphonia, hoarseness
Oropharyngeal fungal
infections
Headache
Sore throat
Nasal congestion, cold
symptoms
Nausea, vomiting, diarrhea
Unpleasant taste, upset
stomach

Nursing Considerations
Used in chronic asthma
treatment, seasonal or
perennial rhinitis
Onset: few days
Use regular peak flow
monitoring to determine
respiratory status
Rx; Preg Cat C

FLUTICASONE
(floo-<u>ti</u>-ka-sone)
(Flonase)

• •

MOMETASONE
(moe-<u>met</u>-a-sone)
(Nasonex)

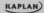

Side Effects
Dysphonia, hoarseness
Oropharyngeal fungal infections
Headache
Sore throat
Nasal congestion, cold symptoms
Nausea, vomiting, diarrhea
Unpleasant taste, upset stomach

Nursing Considerations
Used in chronic asthma treatment, seasonal or perennial rhinitis
Nasal spray onset within 2 days, peak 1–2 weeks
Use regular peak flow monitoring to determine respiratory status
Rx; Preg Cat C

• •

Side Effects
Dysphonia, hoarseness
Oropharyngeal fungal infections
Headache
Sore throat
Nasal congestion, cold symptoms
Nausea, vomiting, diarrhea
Unpleasant taste, upset stomach

Nursing Considerations
Used in chronic asthma treatment, seasonal or perennial rhinitis
Nasal spray: onset few days, peak up to 3 weeks
Use regular peak flow monitoring to determine respiratory status
Rx; Preg Cat C

TRIAMCINOLONE
(trye-am-<u>sin</u>-oh-lone)
(Nasocort spray, Amcort)

• •

ACETAMINOPHEN
(a-seat-a-<u>mee</u>-noe-fen)
(Tylenol)

Side Effects

Dysphonia, hoarseness

Oropharyngeal fungal infections

Headache

Sore throat

Nasal congestion, cold symptoms

Nausea, vomiting, diarrhea

Unpleasant taste, upset stomach

Nursing Considerations

Used in chronic asthma treatment, seasonal or perennial rhinitis

Nasal spray: onset few days, peak 3–4 days

PO/IM: peak 1–2 hours

Use regular peak flow monitoring to determine respiratory status

Rx; Preg Cat C

• •

Side Effects

Anemia (long-term use)

Liver and kidney failure (high prolonged doses)

Nursing Considerations

Treatment of mild pain or fever

PO: onset less than 1 hour, peak 1/2–2 hours, duration 4–6 hours

Rectal: onset slow, peak 1–2 hours, duration 3–4 hours

Take crushed or whole with full glass of water

Can give with food or milk to decrease GI upset

Signs of chronic poisoning: rapid, weak pulse, dyspnea, cold, clammy extremities

Signs of chronic overdose: bleeding, bruising, malaise, fever, sore throat

OTC; Preg Cat B

ASPIRIN
(<u>as</u>-pir-in)

• •

CELECOXIB
(sel-eh-<u>cox</u>-ib)

(Celebrex)

Side Effects

Nausea, vomiting
Rash

Nursing Considerations

Management of mild to
moderate pain or fever,
transient ischemic attacks,
prophylaxis of MI, ischemic
stroke, angina
PO: onset 15–30 minutes,
peak 1–2 hours, duration
4–6 hours
Rectal: onset slow, 20–60%
absorbed if retained
2–4 hours
With long-term use, check
for liver damage: dark
urine, clay-colored stools,
yellowing of skin and sclera,
itching, abdominal pain,
fever, diarrhea
For arthritis, give 30
minutes before exercise;
may take 2 weeks before full
effect is felt
Discard tablets if vinegar-
like smell
Do not give to children or
teens with flulike symptoms
or chickenpox; Reye's syndrome may develop
OTC; Preg Cat C

• •

Side Effects

Recent research shows
increased risk of heart attack or stroke
Serious skin reactions
and intestinal problems
(bleeding ulcers) can occur
without warning
Fatigue, anxiety, depression,
nervousness
Nausea, vomiting, anorexia,
dry mouth, constipation

Nursing Considerations

Also in category of
Nonsteroidal Anti-inflam-
matories
Management of acute,
chronic arthritis pain and
primary dysmenorrhea pain
relief
Can take without regard to
meals
Increasing doses does not
increase effectiveness
Do not take if allergic to
sulfonamides, aspirin, or
NSAIDs, caution with any
Hx of drug allergies
Rx; Preg Cat C for first and
second trimester; Preg Cat
D for third trimester

IBUPROFEN
(eye-byoo-<u>proe</u>-fen)
(Motrin, Advil)

CODEINE
(<u>koe</u>-deen)

Side Effects
Headache
Nausea, anorexia
GI bleeding
Blood dyscrasias

Nursing Considerations
Treatment of rheumatoid arthritis, osteoarthritis, primary dysmenorrhea, gout, dental pain, musculo-skeletal disorders, fever
Onset: 1/2 hour, peak 1–2 hours
Contact clinician if ringing or roaring in ears, which may indicate toxicity
Contact clinician if changes in urinary pattern, increased weight, edema, increased pain in joints, fever, blood in urine, which may indicate kidney damage
Use sunscreen to prevent photosensitivity
Avoid use with ASA, NSAIDs, and alcohol, which may precipitate GI bleeding
OTC/Rx; Preg Cat B

• •

Side Effects
Drowsiness, sedation
Nausea, vomiting, anorexia
Respiratory depression
Constipation
Orthostatic hypotension

Nursing Considerations
Treatment of moderate to severe pain, nonproductive cough
PO: onset 30–45 minutes, peak 60–120 minutes, duration 4–6 hours
IM/subQ: onset 10–30 min-utes, peak 30–60 minutes, duration 4–6 hours
Do not give if respirations are less than 12 per minute
Avoid use with alcohol, other CNS depressants
Withdrawal symptoms may occur: nausea, vomiting, cramps, fever, faintness, anorexia
Physical dependency may result from long-term use
Rx; Schedule C-II, III, IV, V (depends on route); Preg Cat C

HYDROCODONE BITARTRATE & ACETAMINOPHEN
(hi-dro-<u>ko</u>-doan)
(Lortabs)

• •

HYDROMORPHONE
(hye-droe-<u>mor</u>-foan)
(Dilaudid)

Side Effects
- Dizziness
- Drowsiness
- Constipation
- Nausea
- Vomiting

Nursing Considerations
Used for relief of moderate to moderately severe pain
Use with CNS depressants and/or alcohol may result in additive CNS depression
May be habit-forming
Avoid alcohol during treatment
Use with caution in patients with pulmonary considerations
Rx; Schedule C-III; Preg Cat C

• •

Side Effects
- Drowsiness, sedation
- Nausea, vomiting, anorexia
- Respiratory depression
- Constipation, cramps
- Orthostatic hypotension
- Confusion, headache
- Rash

Nursing Considerations
Treatment of moderate to severe pain, nonproductive cough
PO: onset 15–30 minutes, peak 30–60 minutes, duration 4–6 hours
IM: onset 15 minutes, peak 30–60 minutes, duration 4–5 hours

IV: onset 10–15 minutes, peak 15–30 minutes, duration 2–3 hours
SubQ: onset 15 minutes, peak 30–90 minutes, duration 4 hours
Rectal: duration 6–8 hours
Do not give if respirations are less than 12 per minute
Avoid use with alcohol, other CNS depressants
Withdrawal symptoms may occur: nausea, vomiting, cramps, fever, faintness, anorexia
Physical dependency may result from long-term use
Rx; Schedule C-II; Preg Cat C

MEPERIDINE
(me-<u>per</u>-i-deen)
(Demerol)

· ·

METHADONE
(<u>meth</u>-a-doan)

Side Effects

Drowsiness, sedation
Respiratory depression
Euphoria
Orthostatic hypotension
Confusion, headache

Nursing Considerations

Management of moderate to severe pain, pre-op sedation, post-op and OB analgesia
PO: onset 10–15 minutes, peak 30–60 minutes, duration 2–4 hours (usually 3)
IM: onset 10–15 minutes, peak 30–50 minutes, duration 2–4 hours (usually 3)
IV: onset less than 5 minutes, peak 5–7 minutes, duration 2–4 hours (usually 3)
SubQ: onset 10–15 minutes, peak 30–50 minutes, duration 2–4 hours (usually 3)
Do not give if respirations are less than 12 per minute
Avoid use with alcohol, other CNS depressants
Withdrawal symptoms may occur: nausea, vomiting, cramps, fever, faintness, anorexia
Physical dependency may result from long-term use
Rx; Schedule C-II; Preg Cat C

• •

Side Effects

Drowsiness, sedation
Nausea, vomiting, anorexia
Respiratory depression
Constipation, cramps
Orthostatic hypotension
Confusion, headache
Rash

Nursing Considerations

Relief of pain, detoxification/maintenance of narcotic addiction
PO: onset 30–60 minutes, peak 30–60 minutes, duration 4–6 hours (with continuous dosing, duration of action may increase to 22 to 48 hours)
IM: onset 10–20 minutes, peak 60–120 minutes, duration 4–5 hours (with continuous dosing, duration of action may increase to 22 to 48 hours)
IV: onset peak 15–30 minutes, duration 3–4 hours
Do not give if respirations are less than 12 per minute
Avoid use with alcohol, other CNS depressants
Withdrawal symptoms may occur: nausea, vomiting, cramps, fever, faintness, anorexia
Physical dependency may result from long-term use
Rx; Schedule C-II; Preg Cat C

MORPHINE
(<u>mor</u>-feen)
(MS Contin)

• •

OXYCODONE
(ox-i-<u>koe</u>-doan)
(Oxy Contin; with aspirin: Percodan, with acetaminophen: Percoset)

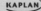

Side Effects
Respiratory depression
Sedation
Euphoria
Orthostatic hypotension

Nursing Considerations
Management of severe pain
Continuous dosing is more
effective than prn; may be
given by patient controlled
analgesia (PCA)
PO: onset 15–60 minutes,
peak 30–60 minutes,
duration 3–6 hours
IM: onset 10–15 minutes,
peak 30–50 minutes, duration
2–4 hours (usually 3)
IV: onset less than 5 minutes,
peak 18 minutes, duration
3–6 hours
SubQ: onset 10–15 minutes,
peak 30–50 minutes, dura-
tion 2–4 hours (usually 3)
Withdrawal symptoms may
occur: nausea, vomiting,
cramps, fever, faintness,
anorexia
Physical dependency may
result from long-term use
Rx; Schedule C-II; Preg
Cat C

· ·

Side Effects
Drowsiness, sedation
Nausea, vomiting, anorexia
Respiratory depression
Constipation, cramps
Orthostatic hypotension
Confusion, headache
Rash
Euphoria

Nursing Considerations
Management of moderate to
severe pain
PO: peak 30–60 minutes,
duration 4–6 hours
Controlled release: peak
3–4 minutes, duration
12 hours
Do not give if respirations
are less than 12 per minute
Avoid use with alcohol,
other CNS depressants
Withdrawal symptoms may
occur: nausea, vomiting,
cramps, fever, faintness,
anorexia
Physical dependency may
result from long-term use
Rx; Schedule C-II; Preg Cat B

PROPOXYPHENE
(proe-<u>pox</u>-i-feen)
**(Darvon, Darvocet-N
(propoxyphene with acetominophen))**

• •

TRAMADOL
(<u>trah</u>-<u>mah</u>-dole)
**(Ultram, Ultram ER, Ultracet
(tramadol with acetominophen))**

Side Effects
Drowsiness, sedation
Nausea, vomiting, anorexia
Respiratory depression
Constipation, cramps
Orthostatic hypotension
Confusion, headache
Rash

Nursing Considerations
Management of mild to
moderate pain
PO: onset 30–60 minutes,
peak 120 minutes, duration
4–6 hours
Low schedule rating for
misuse potential, addiction
liability
Do not use in patients with
suicidal tendencies
Avoid use with alcohol,
other CNS depressants
Withdrawal symptoms may
occur: nausea, vomiting,
cramps, fever, faintness,
anorexia
Physical dependency may
result from long-term use
with high doses
Rx; Schedule C-IV; Preg
Cat C

Side Effects
Dizziness, drowsiness,
sedation
Insomnia
Headache
Nervousness, agitation
Uncontrollable shaking,
muscle tightness
Changes in mood

Nursing Considerations
Management of moderate to
moderately severe pain
Notify prescriber of
significant symptoms: seizures; sores in mouth, nose
or throat; flu-like symp-
toms; hives; rash; difficulty
swallowing or breathing;
hallucinations
Sudden discontinuation
may cause withdrawal
symptoms: nervousness,
panic, sweating, insomnia
Rx; not a controlled
substance; Preg Cat C

HEPARIN
(<u>hep</u>-a-rin)

• •

WARFARIN
(<u>war</u>-far-in)
(Coumadin)

Side Effects

Can produce hemorrhage from any body site (10%)
Tissue irritation/pain at injection site
Anemia
Thrombocytopenia
Fever

Nursing Considerations

Prophylaxis and treatment of thromboembolic disorders. In very low doses (10–100 units) to maintain patency of IV catheters (heparin flush)
Therapeutic PPT @ 1.5–2.5 times the control without signs of hemorrhage
IV: peak 5 minutes, duration 2–6 hours
Injection: give deep SubQ; never IM (danger of hematoma), onset 20–60 minutes, duration 8–12 hours
Antidote: protamine sulfate within 30 minutes
Signs of hemorrhage: bleeding gums, nosebleed, unusual bleeding, black, tarry stools, hematuria, fall in hematocrit or blood pressure, guaiac-positive stools
Avoid ASA-containing products and NSAIDs
Wear medical information tag
Rx; Preg Cat C

• •

Side Effects

Hemorrhage
Diarrhea
Rash
Fever

Nursing Considerations

Management of pulmonary emboli, deep-vein thrombosis, MI, atrial dysrhythmias, postcardiac valve replacement
Therapeutic PT @ 1.5–2.5 times the control, INR @ 2.0–3.0
Onset: 12–24 hours, peak 1 1/2 to 3 days; duration: 3 to 5 days
Antidote: vitamin K, whole blood, plasma
Avoid foods high in Vitamin K: many green leafy vegetables
Do not interchange brands; potencies may not be equivalent
Avoid ASA-containing products and NSAIDs
Wear medical information tag
Rx; Preg Cat X

CARBAMAZEPINE
(kar-ba-<u>maz</u>-e-peen)
(Tegretol, Tegretol XR)

• •

DIVALPROEX SODIUM
(dye-<u>val</u>-proe-ex)
(Depakote, Depokote ER)

Side Effects
Myelosuppression
Dizziness, drowsiness
Ataxia
Diplopia, rash
Photosensitivity

Nursing Considerations
Management of seizures,
trigeminal neuralgia, diabetic neuropathy
Avoid driving and other
activities requiring alertness
the first 3 days
Monitor blood levels, CBC
regularly, esp. during first
2 months; periodic eye exams
Take with food or milk to
decrease GI upset; tablets
(nonextended release) may
be crushed, extended release
capsules may be opened,
mixed with juice or soft
food
Urine may turn pink to
brown
Avoid abrupt withdrawal;
discontinue gradually
Avoid use with alcohol,
other CNS depressants
Rx; Preg Cat C

• •

Side Effects
Sedation, drowsiness,
dizziness
Mental status and
behavioral changes
Nausea, vomiting, constipa-
tion, diarrhea, heartburn
Prolonged bleeding time

Nursing Considerations
Management of seizures,
manic episodes associated
with bipolar disorder (delayed release only), migraine
prophylaxis (delayed and
extended release only)
Take with or immedi-
ately after meals to lessen
GI upset
Swallow tablets or capsules
whole (no crushing, chewing)
Avoid abrupt withdrawal
after long-term use; discontinue gradually to prevent
convulsions
Monitor blood levels,
platelets, bleeding time, and
liver function tests
Delayed release products:
peak blood level 3–5 hours,
duration 12–24 hours
Extended release products:
Onset 2–4 days, peak blood
level 7–14 hours, duration
24 hours
Wear medical information
tag
Rx; Preg Cat D

GABAPENTIN
(gab-ah-<u>pen</u>-tin)
(Neurontin)

• •

LAMOTRIGINE
(lah-<u>moe</u>-tri-jeen)
(Lamictal)

Side Effects
- Drowsiness
- Ataxia
- Diplopia
- Rhinitis
- Constipation

Nursing Considerations
Used for management of seizures and postherpetic neuralgia

Do not take within 2 hours of antacid

Avoid abrupt withdrawal after long-term use; discontinue gradually over a week to prevent convulsions

Give without regard to meals; can open capsules and put in juice or applesauce

Do not crush or chew capsules

Use caution with hazardous activities

Wear medical information tag

Rx; Preg Cat C

• •

Side Effects
- Ataxia, dizziness
- Headache
- Nausea, vomiting, anorexia
- Diplopia, blurred vision
- Abdominal pain
- Dysmenorrhea

Nursing Considerations
Used for management of seizures

In pediatric patients, stop at first sign of rash; all patients should notify clinician of rashes

Take divided doses with meals or just after to decrease adverse effects

Use caution with hazardous activities until stabilized

Avoid abrupt withdrawal; stop gradually to prevent increase in frequency of seizures

Wear medical information tag

Rx; Preg Cat C

PHENOBARBITAL
(fee-noe-<u>bar</u>-bi-tal)
(Luminal)

• •

PHENYTOIN
(<u>fen</u>-i-toyn)
(Dilantin)

Side Effects
Drowsiness, lethargy, rash
GI upset
Initially constricts pupils
Respiratory depression
Ataxia

Nursing Considerations
Management of epilepsy,
febrile seizures in children,
sedation, insomnia
IV: slow rate—
resuscitation equipment
should be available
IM: inject deep into large
muscle mass to prevent
tissue sloughing; can give
subQ, onset 10–30 minutes
PO: onset 20–60 minutes,
peak 8–12 hours, duration
6–10 hours
Use caution with hazardous
activities until stabilized;
drowsiness usually
diminishes after initial
weeks of therapy
Nystagmus may indicate
early toxicity
Long-term use withdrawal
symptoms: vomiting, sweating, abdominal muscle
cramps, tremors, and pos-
sibly convulsions
Vitamin D supplements are
indicated for long-term use
Rx; Schedule C-IV; Preg
Cat D

• •

Side Effects
Drowsiness, ataxia
Nystagmus
Blurred vision
Hirsutism
Lethargy
GI upset
Gingival hypertrophy

Nursing Considerations
Management of seizures,
migraines, trigeminal
neuralgia, Bell's palsy
PO: Take divided doses,
with or immediately after
meals, to decrease adverse
effects
May color urine and sweat
pink/red/brown
IV administration may lead
to cardiac arrest—have
resuscitation equipment
available; never mix in IV
with any other drug or
dextrose
Avoid abrupt withdrawal to
prevent convulsions
Do not use antacids or
antidiarrheals within
2 hours of med
Use caution with hazardous
activities until stabilized
Folic acid supplements are
indicated for long-term use
Wear medical information
tag
Rx; Preg Cat C

PREGABALIN
(pree-<u>gab</u>-<u>ah</u>-lin)
(Lyrica)

· ·

TOPIRAMATE
(toh-<u>pire</u>-ah-mate)
(Topamax)

Side Effects

Tiredness, dizziness
Headache
Dry mouth
Nausea, vomiting,
constipation, gas, bloating
Elevated mood
Confusion, forgetfulness

Nursing Considerations

Treatment of epileptic
seizures, neuropathic pain
for people with diabetes,
shingles, fibromyalgia
Avoid use of alchohol. May
increase drowsiness.
May be habit forming.
Withdrawal symptoms, such
as insomnia or seizures, if
sudden discontinuation.
Diabetics should pay at-
tention to skin condition,
and report sores, redness or
other skin problems.
Contact prescriber if
changes in eyesight, chest
pain or wheezing
Rx; Preg Cat C

• •

Side Effects

Dizziness, drowsiness,
fatigue
Impaired concentration/
memory
Nervousness, speech
problems
Nausea, weight loss
Vision problems
Ataxia
Photosensitivity

Nursing Considerations

Used for management of
seizures
Give without regard to
meals; can open capsules
and put in juice or applesauce
Avoid abrupt withdrawal
after long-term use; discontinue gradually to prevent
seizures and status epilep-
ticus
Use caution with hazardous
activities until stabilized
Increase fluid intake to
prevent formation of kidney
stones
Stop drug immediately if
eye problems; could lead to
permanent loss of vision
Use sunscreen and protec-
tive clothing to prevent
photosensitivity
Wear medical information
tag
Rx; Preg Cat C

VALPROATE, VALPROIC ACID
(val-<u>proe</u>-ate, val-<u>proe</u>-ic <u>as</u>-id)
(Depacon, Depakene)

• •

GENTAMICIN
(jen-ta-<u>mye</u>-sin)
(Garamycin)

Side Effects

Sedation, drowsiness, dizziness

Mental status and behavioral changes

Nausea, vomiting, constipation, diarrhea, heartburn

Prolonged bleeding time

Nursing Considerations

Used for management of seizures

Avoid abrupt withdrawal after long-term use; discontinue gradually to prevent convulsions

Monitor blood levels, platelets, bleeding time, and liver function tests

Duration of anticonvulsant effect: 6–24 hours (varies with age)

Rx; Preg Cat D

- -

Side Effects

Use during pregnancy can result in bilateral congenital deafness

Ototoxicity cranial nerve VIII

Nephrotoxicity

Allergic reaction: fever, difficulty breathing, rash

Nursing Considerations

Treatment of severe systemic infections of CNS, respiratory, GI, urinary tract, bone, skin, soft tissues, acute PID

IV over 1/2 to 1 hr; IM by deep, slow injection, never subQ

Careful monitoring of blood levels

Check peak—2 hours after med given

Check trough—at time of dose/prior to med

Monitor for signs of superinfection (diarrhea, URI, coated tongue)

Immediately report hearing or balance problems

Encourage fluids to 8–10 glasses/day

Rx; Preg Cat C

AMPHOTERICIN B
(am-foe-<u>ter</u>-i-sin)
(Fungizone)

• •

FLUCONAZOLE
(flew-<u>kon</u>-uh-zol)
(Diflucan)

Side Effects

Blood, kidney, heart, liver abnormalities
GI upset
Hypokalemia-induced muscle pain
CNS disturbances, inefficient hearing
Skin irritation and thrombosis if IV infiltrates

Nursing Considerations

Treatment of histoplasmosis, skin infections, septicemia, meningitis in HIV patients
Monitor vital signs; report fever or change in function, especially nervous system
Check for hypokalemia
Meticulous care and observation of injection site
Potential benefits must be balanced against serious side effects
Rx; Preg Cat B

• • • • • • • • • • • • • • • • • • • •

Side Effects

Nausea
Headache
Abdominal pain
Diarrhea
Taste distortion

Nursing Considerations

Used to treat vaginal, esophageal, or systemic candidiasis
Prothrombin time is increased after warfarin usage
Take missed dose as soon as noticed, but do not double dose
Reduces metabolism of tolbutamide, glyburide, and glipizide, so blood glucose levels should be monitored more closely in diabetics
Rx; Preg Cat C

HYDROZYCHLOROQUINE
(hye-drox-ee-<u>klor</u>-oh-kwin)
(Plaquenil)

• •

QUININE SULFATE
(<u>kwye</u>-nine sul-fate)

Side Effects
Eye disturbances
Nausea, vomiting
Anorexia

Nursing Considerations
Management of malaria,
lupus erythematosus, rheumatoid arthritis
Peak 1–2 hours
Take at the same time each
day to maintain blood level
For malaria, prophylaxis
should be started 2 weeks
before exposure and con-
tinue for 4–6 weeks after
leaving exposure area
Rx; Preg Cat C

• •

Side Effects
Eye disturbances
Nausea, vomiting
Anorexia

Nursing Considerations
Treatment of malaria,
nocturnal leg cramps
Peak 1–3 hours
Take at the same time each
day to maintain blood level
Avoid OTC cold meds, tonic
water
OTC/Rx; Preg Cat X

METRONIDAZOLE
(me-troe-<u>ni</u>-da-zole)
(Flagyl, Flagyl ER)

• •

ISONIAZID
(eye-soe-<u>nye</u>-a-zid)
(INH)

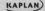

Side Effects
  Headache
  Dizziness
  Nausea, vomiting, diarrhea
  Abdominal cramps
  Metallic taste

Nursing Considerations
  Treatment of a wide variety
  of infections, including
  trichomoniasis and giardiasis
  IV: immediate onset, PO:
  peak 1–2 hours
  Urine may turn dark-red-
  dish brown
  Avoid hazardous activities
  Treatment of both partners
  is necessary in trichomoniasis
  Do not drink alcohol or
  preparations containing
  alcohol during and 48 hours
  after use, disulfiram-like
  reaction can occur
  Rx; Preg Cat B

• •

Side Effects
  Peripheral neuropathy
  Liver damage

Nursing Considerations
  Prevention and treatment
  of TB
  PO/IM: onset rapid, peak
  1–2 hours, duration up to
  24 hours
  Contact clinician if signs of
  hepatitis: yellow eyes and
  skin, nausea, vomiting,
  anorexia, dark urine, unusual
  tiredness, or weakness
  Contact clinician if signs
  of peripheral neuropathy:
  numbness, tingling, or
  weakness
  Rx; Preg Cat C

ACYCLOVIR
(ay-<u>sye</u>-kloe-ver)
(Zovirax)

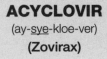

OSELTAMIVIR PHOSPHATE
(oh-sul-<u>tamm</u>-eh-vere <u>foss</u>-fate)
(Tamiflu)

Side Effects
Headache
Blood dyscrasias

Nursing Considerations
Treatment of herpes,
varicella
IV: onset immediate, peak
immediate
PO: absorbed minimally,
onset unknown, peak 1 1/2
hours
Do not break, crush, or
chew capsules
PO: Take without regard
to meals with a full glass of
water
If dose is missed, take as
soon as remembered, up to
1 hour before next dose
Contact clinician if sore
throat, fever and fatigue,
could be signs of superinfection
Rx; Preg Cat B

Side Effects
Nausea
Vomiting

Nursing Considerations
Used as prophylaxis in
adults for influenza, including Avian Bird Flu
Used to treat uncomplicated
acute flu symptoms in
patients symptomatic for
less than 2 days
Should not be used as a
substitute for influenza
vaccinations
May be taken without
regard to meals
Rx; Preg Cat C

VALACYCLOVIR HCL
(val-uh-<u>sy</u>-kloe-veer)
(Valtrex)

● ●

ZIDOVUDINE
(zye-<u>doe</u>-vue-deen)
(AZT, Retrovir)

Side Effects

Nausea
Vomiting
Headache
Abdominal cramps

Nursing Considerations

For the treatment of genital
Herpes, Herpes Zoster
(shingles), Herpes Labialis
(cold sores)
Patients should drink plenty
of fluids during treatment
Avoid sexual contact when
lesions are visible
Use with caution in preg-
nancy and nursing mothers
Rx; Preg Cat B

• •

Side Effects

Fever, headache, malaise
Dizziness
Insomnia
Dyspepsia
Nausea, vomiting, diarrhea
Anorexia
Rash

Nursing Considerations

Management of HIV infec-
tions and prevention of HIV
following needlestick
GI upset and insomnia
resolve after 3–4 weeks
PO: peak 1/2–1 1/2 hours
Rx; Preg Cat C

CEFADROXIL, CEPHALEXIN
(sef-a-<u>drox</u>-ill, sef-a-<u>lex</u>-in)
(Duricef, Keflex/Keflet)

• •

Anti-Infectives
CEPHALOSPORINS, SECOND GENERATION

CEFACLOR, CEFOTETAN, CEFOXITIN, CEFPROZIL, CEFUROXIME
(<u>sef</u>-a-klor, sef-oh-<u>tee</u>-tan, se-<u>fox</u>-i-tin,
sef-<u>proe</u>-zill, sef-yoo-<u>rox</u>-eem)
**(Ceclor/Ceclor CD, Cefotan,
Mefoxin, Cefzil, Ceftin)**

Side Effects
Diarrhea

Nursing Considerations
Treatment of infections:
respiratory tract, skin and
bone, otitis media, tonsil-
litis, UTIs, endocarditis,
peritonitis
Avoid alcohol
Eat yogurt or buttermilk to
maintain intestinal flora
Take for 10-14 days to prevent superinfection
Rx; Preg Cat B

● ●

Side Effects
Diarrhea

Nursing Considerations
Treatment of a wide range of
infections: respiratory tract,
skin, joint and bone, otitis
media, pharyngitis/tonsil-
litis, UTIs, peritonitis, GYN
and gonococcal, meningi-
tis, septicemia, secondary
bacterial infection of acute
bronchitis, acute bacterial
exacerbation of chronic
bronchitis, acute sinusitis
Can be used for surgical
prophylaxis
Avoid alcohol
Eat yogurt or buttermilk to
maintain intestinal flora
Take for 10–14 days to
prevent superinfection
Rx; Preg Cat B

CEFDINIR, CEFEPIME, CEFOPERAZONE, CEFOTAXIME, CEFPODOXIME

(<u>sef</u>-dih-ner, <u>sef</u>-e-peem, sef-oh-<u>per</u>-a-zone, sef-oh-<u>taks</u>-eem, sef-poe-<u>docks</u>-eem)

(Omincef, Maxipime, Cefobid, Claforan, Vantin)

• •

Anti-Infectives
FLUOROQUINOLONES

CIPROFLOXACIN

(sip-ro-<u>flocks</u>-a-sin)

(Cipro)

Side Effects
Nausea, vomiting, anorexia
Diarrhea

Nursing Considerations
Treatment of infections:
respiratory tract, skin and
bone, otitis media, UTIs,
peritonitis, GYN and STDs,
meningitis, septicemia,
bacteremia, acute bacterial
exacerbation of chronic
bronchitis
Avoid alcohol
Eat yogurt or buttermilk to
maintain intestinal flora
Take for 10-14 days to prevent superinfection
Rx; Preg Cat B

• •

Side Effects
Seizures
Nausea, vomiting, diarrhea,
abdominal distress, flatulence
Rash
Photosensitivity

Nursing Considerations
Treatment of infection
caused by E. coli and other
bacteria, chronic bacterial
prostatis, acute sinusitis,
postexposure inhalation
anthrax
Contraindicated in children
less than 18 years of age
Take 2 hours after meals or
2 hours before an antacid or
iron preparation
Take at equal intervals
around the clock
Avoid caffeine
Encourage fluids to 8–10
glasses/day
Rx; Preg Cat C

VANCOMYCIN
(van-koe-<u>mye</u>-sin)
(Lyphocin, Vancocin, Vancoled)

. . . .

CLINDAMYCIN
(klin-da-<u>my</u>-sin)
(Cleocin HCl, Cleocin Phosphate for IM)

Side Effects
  Liver damage

Nursing Considerations
  Treatment of resistant staph
  infections, colitis, staph
  enterocolitis, endocarditis
  prophylaxis for dental procedures (used for c. difficile)
  PO: poor absorption
  IV: peak 5 minutes, duration
  12–24 hours
  Give antihistamine if "red
  man syndrome": decreased
  blood pressure, flushing of
  face and neck
  Contact clinician if signs of
  superinfection: sore throat,
  fever, fatigue
  Rx; Preg Cat C

· ·

Side Effects
  Nausea, vomiting, diarrhea
  Abdominal pain
  Vaginitis

Nursing Considerations
  Treatment of infections
  caused by staph, strep, and
  other organisms
  PO: peak 45 minutes,
  duration 6 hours
  IM: peak 3 hours, duration
  8–12 hours
  Rx; Preg Cat B

KAPLAN

AZITHROMYCIN
(ay-zi-thro-<u>my</u>-sin)
(Zithromax)

· ·

CLARITHROMYCIN
(klair-<u>ith</u>-row-my-sin)
(Biaxin, Biaxin XL)

Side Effects
  Nausea, vomiting, diarrhea

Nursing Considerations
  Treatment of mild to
  moderate infections of
  the respiratory tract, skin,
  nongonoccocal urethritis,
  cervicitis, acute pharyngi-
  tis/tonsillitis, community
  acquired pneumonia
  PO: rapid onset, peak
  2.5–3.2 hours, duration
  24 hours
  IV: rapid onset, peak end of
  infusion, duration 24 hours
  PO: don't take with antacids;
  can take with or without
  food

Monitor for signs of superinfection (diarrhea, perineal
itching, oral ulcers)
If treated for nongonococ-
cal urethritis or cervicitis,
sexual partners also need
treatment
Rx; Preg Cat B

• •

Side Effects
  Nausea
  Diarrhea
  Dyspepsia
  Taste abnormalities

Nursing Considerations
  Used for respiratory
  infections
  Treatment may be 7–14 days
  depending on organism and
  extent of infection
  Medication should be taken
  with food
  Be aware of possible increase in theophylline and
  carbamazepine levels
  Rx; Preg Cat C

ERYTHROMYCIN
(eh-rith-roe-<u>mye</u>-sin)
(Ery-Tab, Erythrocin)

• •

AMOXICILLIN, AMPICILLIN, PENICILLIN
(ah-mox-ih-<u>sill</u>-in, am-pih-<u>sill</u>-in, pen-i-<u>sill</u>-in)
(Amoxil, Omnipen, Bicillin, Wycillin)

Side Effects

Abdominal cramps
Pain at injection site
Nausea, vomiting, diarrhea

Nursing Considerations

Treatment of infections, including chlamydia, syphilis
PO: Give 1 hr ac/2 hr pc with full glass H_2O (avoid citrus juice); some formulations can be given without regard to meals
PO: onset 1 hour, peak up to 4 hours, duration 6–12 hours
IV: onset rapid, peak end of infusion, duration 6–12 hours

Take at equal intervals around the clock
Can be used in patients with compromised renal function
Monitor for signs of super-infection (diarrhea, perineal itching, oral ulcers)
Rx; Preg Cat B

• •

Side Effects

Allergic reactions: fever, difficulty breathing, skin rash
Renal, hepatic, hematologic abnormalities
Nausea, vomiting, diarrhea

Nursing Considerations

Treatment of respiratory infections, scarlet fever, otitis media, pneumonia, skin and soft tissue infections, gonorrhea
Take careful history of penicillin reaction; observe for 20 minutes post IM injection
PO for penicillin and ampicillin: Take 1 hour before meals or 2 hours after meals to reduce gastric acid destruction of drug. Not true for amoxicillin
Take equally divided doses around the clock
Continue medication for entire time prescribed, even if symptoms resolve
Check for hypersensitivity to other drugs, especially cephalosporins
Rx; Preg Cat B

SULFISOXAZOLE
(sul-fi-<u>sox</u>-a-zole)
(Gantrisin)

· ·

TRIMETHOPRIM-
SULFAMETHOXAZOLE
(trye-<u>meth</u>-oh-prim-sul-fa-meth-<u>ox</u>-a-zole)
(Bactrim, Septra)

Side Effects
Headache
Nausea, vomiting, diarrhea
Allergic rash
Urinary crystallization
Photosensitivity

Nursing Considerations
Treatment of urinary tract, systemic infections, chancroid, trachoma, toxoplasmosis, acute otitis media, malaria (adjunctive therapy), meningitis, eye infections
PO: full glass H_2O
Monitor I and 0, force fluids
Rx; Preg Cat C

• •

Side Effects
Hypersensitivity reaction
Blood dyscrasias
Stop at first sign of skin rash
Photosensitivity

Nursing Considerations
Treatment of urinary tract, chancroid, acute otitis media, acute and chronic prostatitis, shigellosis, pneumoonitis, chronic bronchitis, traveler's diarrhea
PO: with full glass H_2O; if upset stomach occurs, take with food
PO: Take at equal intervals around the clock
IV solution must be given slowly over 60–90 minutes; flush lines at end of infusion to remove residual
Never administer IM, rapidly IV, or by bolus injection
Encourage fluids to 8–10 glasses/day
Rx; Preg Cat C

DOXYCYCLINE, MINOCYCLINE
(DOX-I-<u>SYE</u>-KLEEN, MI-NOE-<u>SYE</u>-KLEEN)
(Vibramycin, Vibra-Tabs, Minocin)

• •

Anti-Inflammatory Medications
CORTICOSTEROIDS

DEXAMETHASONE
(dex-a-<u>meth</u>-a-sone)
(Decadron, Decadron-LA, Decadron Phosphate)

Side Effects
Photosensitivity
GI upset, diarrhea
Renal, hepatic, hematologic
abnormalities
Dental discoloration of
deciduous (baby) teeth

Nursing Considerations
Treatment of syphilis, chlamydia, gonorrhea, malaria
prophylaxis, periodontitis,
acne
Peak 2–4 hours
If GI symptoms occur,
administer with food
EXCEPT milk products or
other foods high in calcium
(interferes with absorption)

Take with full glass of water,
do NOT take within 1 hour
of bedtime or reclining
Check patient's tongue for
Monilia infection
Discard outdated prescrip-
tions
Avoid prolonged exposure
to direct sunlight, UV light
Avoid during tooth and
early development periods
(4th month prenatal to 8
years of age)
Rx; Preg Cat D

• •

Side Effects
Depression
Flushing, sweating
Hypertension
Nausea, diarrhea
Abdominal distention
Increased appetite

Nursing Considerations
Treatment of inflammation,
allergies, neoplasms, cerebral edema, septic shock,
collagen disorders
PO: Take with food, milk,
antacids
IV: use sodium phosphate
form, not acetate (injection
suspension)
IM: shake suspension well,

give deep into gluteal UOQ,
avoid deltoid, rotate sites
Excessive consumption of
licorice can increase risk of
hypokalemia
Eat food high in protein,
calcium, vitamin D; avoid
sodium
Contact clinician if anorexia,
difficulty breathing, weakness, dizziness
Contact clinician if black/
tarry stools, slow wound
healing, blurred vision,
bruising/bleeding, weight
gain, emotional changes
Wear medical identifica-
tion tag
Rx; Preg Cat C

HYDROCORTISONE
(hy-dro-<u>kor</u>-tih-sone)
(Cortef, Solu-Cortef)

• •

METHYLPREDNISOLONE, PREDNISOLONE
(meth-ill-pred-<u>niss</u>-oh-lone, pred-<u>niss</u>-oh-lone)
(Medrol, Prelone, Cortalone)

Side Effects
Depression
Flushing, sweating
Hypertension
Nausea, diarrhea

Nursing Considerations
Treatment of severe inflammation, septic shock, adrenal insufficiency, ulcerative colitis, collagen disorders
Med masks signs of infection, so check for elevated temperature, WBC count
PO: Take with food, milk, antacids
IM: give deep into gluteal UOQ, avoid deltoid, rotate sites, avoid subQ administration since it may damage tissue
Rectal: for colitis, retain med for 20 minutes, onset 3–5 days
Wear medical identification tag
Rx; Preg Cat C

• •

Side Effects
Peptic ulcer/possible perforation
Hypertension and circulatory problems
Poor wound healing
Depression
Nausea, diarrhea
Abdominal distention

Nursing Considerations
Treatment of severe inflammation, imunosuppression, neoplasms, shock, adrenal insufficiency, management of acute spinal cord injury, collagen disorders
PO: Take with food, milk, antacids
PO: duration 18–36 hours
IM: give deep into gluteal UOQ, avoid deltoid, rotate sites, avoid subQ administration, since it may damage tissue
IM: duration 1–4 weeks
Eat food high in protein, calcium, vitamin D; avoid sodium
Contact clinician if anorexia, difficulty breathing, weakness, dizziness; symptoms may appear during periods of stress or trauma
Contact clinician if black/tarry stools, slow wound healing, blurred vision, bruising/bleeding, weight gain, emotional changes
Wear medical identification tag
Rx; Preg Cat C

Anti-Inflammatory Medications
CORTICOSTEROIDS

PREDNISONE
(<u>pred</u>-ni-sone)
(Cordrol, Deltasone, Predacort)

• •

Anti-Inflammatory Medications
NONSTEROIDAL ANTI-INFLAMMATORIES

NABUMETONE
(nay-<u>boom</u>-eh-tone)
(Refalen)

Side Effects

Peptic ulcer/possible perforation

Depression

Hypertension, circulatory problems

Nausea, diarrhea

Abdominal distention

Nursing Considerations

Treatment of severe inflammation, immunosuppression, neoplasms, multiple sclerosis, collagen disorders, dermatologic disorders

PO: Take with food, milk, antacids

PO: peak 1–2 hours, duration 1–1/2 days

Eat food high in protein, calcium, vitamin D; avoid sodium

Contact clinician if anorexia, difficulty breathing, weakness, dizziness; symptoms may appear during periods of stress or trauma

Contact clinician if black/tarry stools, slow wound healing, blurred vision, bruising/bleeding, weight gain, emotional changes

Excessive consumption of licorice can increase risk of hypokalemia

Wear medical identification tag

Rx; Preg Cat C

• •

Side Effects

Abdominal pain

Constipation

Diarrhea

Flatulence

Tinnitus

Edema

Nursing Considerations

Used to manage symptoms of osteoarthritis and rheumatoid arthritis

Take with food or milk

Contraindicated in patients with hypersensitivity to other NSAIDs

Alcohol may increase ulcerogenic effects if used concurrently

May take 2 weeks or more to notice improvement

Rx; Preg Cat C

IBUPROFEN
(eye-byoo-<u>proe</u>-fen)

(Motrin, Advil)

· ·

NAPROXEN
(na-<u>prox</u>-en)

(Naprosyn, Anaprox, Anaprox-DS, EC-Naprosyn, Aleve (OTC))

Side Effects
Headache
Nausea, anorexia
GI bleeding
Blood dyscrasias

Nursing Considerations
Treatment of rheumatoid arthritis, osteoarthritis, primary dysmenorrhea, gout, dental pain, musculoskeletal disorders, fever
Onset: 1/2 hour, peak 1–2 hours,
Contact clinician if blurred vision, ringing or roaring in ears, which may indicate toxicity
Contact clinician if changes in urinary pattern, increased weight, edema, increased pain in joints, fever, blood in urine, which may indicate kidney damage
Full therapeutic effect may take up to 1 month
Avoid use with ASA, NSAIDs, and alcohol, which may precipitate GI bleeding
OTC/Rx; Preg Cat B

• •

Side Effects
GI bleeding
Blood dyscrasias

Nursing Considerations
Management of mild to moderate pain. Treatment of rheumatoid, juvenile, and gouty arthritis, osteoarthritis, primary dysmenorrhea
Patients with asthma, ASA hypersensitivity, or nasal polyps have increased risk of hypersensitivity
Contact clinician if blurred vision, ringing or roaring in ears, which may indicate toxicity
Contact clinician if black stools, flulike symptoms
Contact clinician if changes in urinary pattern, increased weight, edema, increased pain in joints, fever, blood in urine, which may indicate kidney damage
Use sunscreen to prevent photosensitivity
Avoid use with ASA, steroids and alcohol
OTC/Rx; Preg Cat B

CYCLOPHOSPHAMIDE
(sye-kloe-<u>foss</u>-fa-mide)
(Cytoxan, CTX)

• •

DOXORUBICIN
(dox-oh-<u>roo</u>-bih-sin)
(Adriamycin, Doxil, Rubex)

Side Effects
Lowered blood counts
(WBCs, Platelets, RBCs)
Nausea, vomiting, loss of
appetite
Hair loss
Loss of menstrual periods,
decreased sex drive
Bladder irritation
Metallic taste in mouth dur-
ing injection

Nursing Implications
Treatment of lymphomas,
multiple myeloma, leuke-
mias, mycosis fungoides,
retinoblastoma, and ovarian
and breast cancer
Contact prescriber before
having any vaccinations,
such as measles or flu shots
Contact prescriber if severe
mouth blistering or fatigue
Also needing immediate
attention would be painful
urination or
bloody urine, black/tarry
stools and any unusual
bruising or bleeding
Rx; Preg Cat D

• •

Side Effects
Hair loss, mouth sores
Nausea, vomiting
Lowered blood counts
(WBCs, RBCs and platelets)
Damage to heart muscle
Skin damage if drug leaks
out of vein during infusion

Nursing Implications
Treatment of cancers,
including Kaposi's sarcoma
in AIDS
Contact prescriber before
having any vaccinations,
such as measles or flu shots
Contact prescriber if severe
mouth blistering or fatigue.
Also needing immediate
attention would be painful
urination or bloody urine,
unusual bruising or bleeding, pain at injection site,
any change in normal bowel
patterns lasting longer than
2 days
Rx; Preg Cat D

FLUOROURACIL
(flure-oh-<u>yoor</u>-a-sill)
(5-FU, Adrucil)

• •

LETROZOLE
(<u>let</u>-roe-zoal)
(Femara)

Side Effects

Nausea, vomiting, loss of appetite

Thinning or loss of hair

Skin rash and itching, skin darkening

Weakness

Nursing Implications

Treatment of cancers: colon, rectal, breast, stomach, pancreas, ovarian, cervical, bladder

Contact prescriber before having any vaccinations, such as measles or flu shots

Contact prescriber if severe mouth blistering or fatigue. Also needing immediate attention would be painful urination or bloody urine, black/tarry stools, diarrhea, stomach pain and any unusual bruising or bleeding

Rx; Preg Cat D

• •

Side Effects

Hot flashes, night sweats

Nausea, vomiting, diarrhea, anorexia

Muscle, joint or bone pain

Excessive tiredness, muscle weakness, dizziness

Nursing Considerations

Treatment of early breast cancer either right after surgery, radiation and/or chemotherapy or five years after tamoxifen use. Also for breast cancer metastases

Only for post-menopausal women

Since drug may cause or worsen osteoporosis, educate about ways to reduce risk

Contact prescriber if chest pain or difficulty breathing

Rx; Preg Cat D

MERCAPTOPURINE
(mer-kap-toe-<u>pyoor</u>-een)

(6-MP, Leukerin, Mercaleukin, Purinethol)

METHOTREXATE
(meth-oh-<u>trex</u>-ate)

**(Trexall, Rheumatrex, Amethopterin,
MTX, Mexate, Emtexate, Metatrexan,
Methopterin, Folex)**

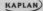

Side Effects
  Low blood counts
  Mouth sores, skin rash, acne
  Nausea
  Abnormal liver function.

Nursing Implications
  Treatment of leukemia,
  many types of autoimmune
  diseases, some anemias,
  multiple sclerosis, myasthenia gravis, ulcerative colitis
  Contact prescriber before
  having any vaccinations,
  such as measles or flu shots
  Contact prescriber if painful
  urination or bloody urine,
  black/tarry stools, diarrhea, stomach pain and any
  unusual bruising or
  Bleeding
  Rx; Preg Cat D

• •

Side Effects
  Abnormal liver function
  tests
  Nausea, vomiting, diarrhea
  Mouth sores, nausea, vomit-
  ing, anorexia, upset stomach
  Alopecia
  Skin and eye sensitivity to
  sunlight
  Anemia

Nursing Implications
  Treatment of cancer,
  mycosis fungoides, pso-
  riasis, rheumatoid arthritis,
  Crohn's disease
  Avoid crowds or people
  with known infections
  Monitor for pulmonary

toxicity, which may manifest
early as a dry, nonproductive cough
Do not take ASA or other
NSAIDs which may cause
GI bleeding
Do not drink alcohol while
taking methotrexate
If for rheumatoid arthritis
treatment, can take 3 to 6
weeks (or longer) for full
effect
Contact prescriber if chest
pain, fainting, vision problems, difficulty speaking or
moving
Rx; Preg Cat X

PACLITAXEL
(<u>pak</u>-lih-tax-ell)
(Onxol, Taxol)

• •

TAMOXIFEN
(ta-mox-i-fen)
(Nolvadex)

Side Effects
Low blood pressure
Shortness of breath
Rash
Loss of hair
Low blood cell counts
Nerve pain

Nursing Implications
Treatment of metatastic
breast and ovarian cancer,
Kaposi's sarcoma, head and
neck cancer, lung cancer,
bladder cancer
Patients take desamethasone
(Decadron) before treat-
ment with paclitaxel
Contact prescriber before
having any vaccinations,
such as measles or flu shots
Contact prescriber if pain,
redness or swelling at the
injection site, change in normal bowel patterns lasting
more than 2 days and any
unusual bruising or bleeding
Rx; Preg Cat D

• •

Side Effects
nausea, vomiting
hot flashes
headache
light-headedness
rash

Nursing Implications
Estrogen antagonist used in
management of advanced
breast cancer in estrogen-
receptor-positive patients
and can be prophylaxis for
women at high risk
To decrease GI upset, take
after antacid, after evening
meal, before bedtime or take
antiemetic 30–60 minutes
ahead

Vaginal bleeding, pruritus,
hot flashes are reversible
after stopping med
Contact prescriber if de-
creased visual acuity, which
may be irreversible
Tumor flare (increase in
tumor size and increased
bone pain) may occur, but
will decrease rapidly; may
take analgesics for pain
Rx; Preg Cat D

THALIDOMIDE
(thah-<u>lih</u>-doe-mide)
(Thalomid)

· ·

VINCRISTINE
(vin-<u>kris</u>-teen)
(Oncovin, Vincasar, Vincrex, Leurocristine)

Side Effects
  Drowsiness, dizziness
  Slower hearbeats
  Photosensitivity

Nursing Implications
  Treatment of primary brain
  malignancies, Kaposi's
  sarcoma, leprosy, lupus
  Contact prescriber if rash,
  fever, numbness, tingling,
  pain or a burning sensation
  in hands or feet
  Alcohol will add to drowsiness side effect. No driving
  or operating machinery
  until effects known
  Cannot give blood or donate
  sperm during treatment
  Rx; Preg Cat X

• •

Side Effects
  Bloating, nausea and vomit-
  ing
  Skin rash
  Temporary loss of hair
  Neurological problems

Nursing Implications
  Treatment of leukemia,
  Hodgkin's disease, non-
  Hodgkin's lymphomas,
  neuroblastoma, rhabdo-
  myosarcoma, Wilms' tumor,
  Kaposi's sarcoma
  Contact prescriber before
  having any vaccinations,
  such as measles or flu shots
  Contact prescriber if severe
  mouth blistering or fatigue.

Also needing immediate attention would be increased,
painful or difficult urination, tingling, numbness or
cramping in the arms or legs
for longer than a few days,
severe abdominal or muclce
cramping, difficulty walk-
ing, talking, or seeing
Rx; Preg Cat D

BENAZEPRIL HCL
(beh-<u>nay</u>-suh-pril)
(Lotesin)

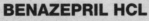

CAPTOPRIL
(<u>kap</u>-toe-pril)
(Capoten)

Side Effects
  Cough
  Headache
  Dizziness
  Angioedema
  Fatigue

Nursing Considerations
  Used to treat hypertension
  Often used in combination
  with thiazide diuretics
  Indomethacin may decrease
  therapeutic effects
  Avoid potassium containing
  salt substitutes because of
  potassium-sparing effect
  Avoid nonprescription
  cough medications unless
  physician directed
  Rx; Preg Cat C

• •

Side Effects
  Dizziness
  Orthostatic hypotension
  Tachycardia
  Bronchospasm, dyspnea,
  cough
  Loss of taste

Nursing Considerations
  Treatment of hypertension,
  CHF, left ventricular dysfunction after MI, diabetic
  neuropathy
  Contact clinician if fever,
  skin rash, sore throat, mouth
  sores, swelling of hands or
  feet, fast or irregular heartbeat, chest pain, or cough
  Take on empty stomach
  1 hour before meals or
  2 hours after; tablets may
  be crushed and mixed with
  juice or soft food for ease of
  swallowing
  Loss of taste might last for
  first 2–3 months, clinical
  concern is interference with
  nutrition
  Avoid changing positions
  (sitting/standing/lying) rapidly,
  especially during the first few
  days, before body adjusts to
  med
  Do not use OTC (cough,
  cold or allergy) meds unless
  directed by clinician
  Avoid potassium supple-
  ments and K salt substitute
  Rx; Preg Cat first trimester
  C; second trimester D

ENALAPRIL MALEATE
(e-<u>nal</u>-a-pril)
(Vasotec)

. . . .

LISINOPRIL
(lye-<u>sin</u>-oh-pril)
(Prinivil, Zestril)

Side Effects
Headache
Dizziness, hypotension
Tachycardia
Tinnitus
Hyperkalemia

Nursing Considerations
Treatment of hypertension, CHF, left ventricular dysfunction
Contact clinician if fever, skin rash, sore throat, mouth sores, swelling of hands or feet, fast or irregular heartbeat, chest pain, or cough
Avoid changing positions (sitting/standing/lying) rapidly, especially during the first few days, before body adjusts to med
Cardiovascular adverse reactions may reoccur
Do not use OTC (cough, cold, or allergy) meds unless directed by clinician
Avoid potassium supplements and potassium salt substitutes
Rx; Preg Cat first trimester C; second trimester D

- - - - - - - - - - - - - - - - - - - -

Side Effects
Headache
Dizziness
Hypotension
Tachycardia
Nausea, vomiting, diarrhea
Fatigue

Nursing Considerations
Treatment of mild to moderate hypertension, systolic CHF, acute MI
Avoid changing positions (lying/sitting/standing) rapidly
May take without regard to food
Avoid high sodium foods (canned soups, lunch meats, cheese)
Avoid high potassium foods (bananas, citrus fruits, raisins)
Rx; Preg Cat first trimester C; second trimester D

DOXAZOSIN MESYLATE
(dox-ay-zoe-sin)
(Cardura)

• •

PRAZOSIN HCL
(pray-zoh-sin)
(Minipress)

Side Effects
  Dizziness
  Headache
  Fatigue, malaise

Nursing Considerations
  Treatment of hypertension,
  benign prostatic hyperplasia
  (BPH)
  Avoid changing positions
  (lying/sitting/standing)
  rapidly
  Can have first dose syncope,
  maintain recumbent for 90
  minutes
  Wear medical identification tag
  Full therapeutic effects may
  require several weeks of
  therapy
  Avoid high sodium foods
  (canned soups, lunch meats,
  cheese)
  Use caution in potentially
  hazardous activities until
  stabilized
  Avoid alcohol, smoking
  Use linked to small pupil
  syndrome during cataract
  surgery
  Rx; Preg Cat C

• •

Side Effects
  Dizziness
  Drowsiness
  Headache
  Nausea, vomiting, diarrhea
  Palpitations

Nursing Considerations
  Treatment of hypertension
  Onset 2 hours, peak 1–3
  hours, duration 6–12 hours
  Can have first dose syncope,
  take the first dose (and any
  increment) at bedtime, do
  not drive for 24 hours
  Full therapeutic effects
  may require 4–6 weeks of
  therapy
  Food may delay absorption
  and minimize side effects
  Avoid changing positions
  (lying/sitting/standing)
  rapidly
  Check with clinician before
  using OTC cold, cough and
  allergy meds
  Rx; Preg Cat C

TERAZOSIN HCL
(ter-<u>ay</u>-zoh-sin)
(Hytrin)

• •

Cardiovascular Medications
ANTI-ANGINALS

ISOSORBIDE DINITRATE,
ISOSORBIDE MONONITRATE
(eye-soe-<u>sor</u>-bide)
(Ismo, Isordil)

Side Effects
 Dizziness
 Headache
 Drowsiness
 Nausea

Nursing Considerations
 Treatment of hypertension,
 benign prostatic hyperplasia
 (BPH)
 Avoid changing positions
 (lying/sitting/standing)
 rapidly
 Can have first dose syncope,
 take the first dose (and any
 increment) at bedtime, do
 not drive or operate ma-
 chinery for 4 hours
 Rx; Preg Cat C

• •

Side Effects
 Dizziness, postural
 hypotension
 Vascular headache, flushing
 Drowsiness
 Nausea

Nursing Considerations
 Treatment/prophylaxis of
 angina pectoris, CHF
 PO: 1 hour before food or
 2 hours after meals for
 maximum absorption, but
 taking with food may reduce
 or eliminate headache
 Chewable tablet: chew well,
 hold in mouth for 2 minutes
 before swallowing
 Sublingual: dissolve under
 tongue, do not eat, drink,
 talk or smoke during use, go
 to ED if pain not relieved in
 15 minutes
 Avoid changing positions
 (lying/sitting/standing)
 rapidly
 Use caution in potentially
 hazardous activities until
 stabilized
 Avoid alcohol, smoking,
 strenuous exercise in hot
 environment
 Wear medical identifica-
 tion tag
 Rx; Preg Cat C

NITROGLYCERIN
(nye-troe-<u>gli</u>-ser-in)
**(Nitro-dur, Transderm-Nitro,
Nitrol/Nitrostat, Nitrotab)**

• •

Cardiovascular Medications
ANTI-ARRHYTHMICS

AMIODARONE HCL
(am-ee-<u>oh</u>-da-rone)
(Cordarone, Pacerone)

Side Effects

Transient headache

Nursing Considerations

Treatment/prophylaxis of angina pectoris; IV used for control of BP during surgery and CHF associated with acute MI

Sustained release: take every 6–12 hours on an empty stomach; onset 20–45 minutes, duration 3–8 hours

Sublingual: patient sitting/lying should let tablet dissolve under tongue and not swallow saliva; onset 1–3 minutes, duration 30 minutes

Spray: hold cannister vertically, spray on tongue, close mouth immediately, not inhale spray; onset 2 minutes, duration 30–60 minutes

IV: use infusion pump and special non-PVC tubing; onset 1–2 minutes, duration 3–5 minutes

Ointment: spread on skin in thin uniform layer; onset 30–60 minutes, duration 2–12 hours

Transdermal: apply to clean hairless area; rotate sites; onset 30–60 minutes, duration 12–24 hours

Go to ED if pain not relieved with 3 tablets in 15 minutes

Wear medical identification tag

Rx; Preg Cat C

• •

Side Effects

Dizziness, fatigue, malaise

Corneal microdeposits

Bradycardia, hypotension

Nausea, vomiting

Anorexia, constipation

Photosensitivity

Neurologic dysfunction

Nursing Considerations

Management of ventricular arrhythmias unresponsive to less toxic agents

IV: continuous cardiac monitoring

Assess for signs of pulmonary toxicity: rales/crackles, decreased breath sounds, pleuritic friction rub, fatigue, dyspnea, cough, pleuritic pain, fever

Neurotoxicity (ataxia, muscle weakness, tingling or numbness in fingers or toes, uncontrolled movements, tremors) common during initial therapy

Side effects may not appear until several days, weeks or years and may persist for several months after stopping med

Teach patient to check radial pulse

Use sunscreen and protective clothing to prevent photosensitivity

Rx; Preg Cat D

LIDOCAINE HCL
(<u>LYE</u>-DOE-KANE)
(Xylocaine)

· ·

PROCAINAMIDE
(proe-<u>kane</u>-a-mide)
(Procanbid, Pronestyl)

Side Effects

- Hypotension, tremors
- Double vision
- Tinnitus
- Confusion, blurred vision
- Drowsiness, dizziness
- Twitching, convulsions
- Respiratory depression/ arrest
- Bradycardia

Nursing Considerations

- Used for premature ventricular contractions
- Give oxygen; have resuscitation equipment available
- IV: use infusion pump; patient on cardiac monitor
- Check BUN, creatinine
- Rx; Preg Cat B

• •

Side Effects

- Hypotension
- Bradycardia
- Fever, rash
- Nausea and vomiting
- Dizziness
- Neutropenia

Nursing Considerations

- Management of life-threatening ventricular dysrhythmias
- IV: use infusion pump; monitor BP q 5–15 minutes; on cardiac monitor; keep patient recumbent
- IV: monitor CBC, blood levels, I&O, daily weight
- PO: best absorption on empty stomach, may take with food to decrease GI upset
- Take at equal intervals around the clock
- Teach patient to check radial pulse
- Avoid caffeine
- Rx; Preg Cat C

QUINIDINE
(<u>kwin</u>-i-deen)
(Quinaglute)

• •

CLONIDINE
(<u>kloe</u>-ni-deen)
**(Catapres patch; Catapres and
Catapres TTS oral tablets)**

Side Effects
- Anemia
- Hypotension
- Headache
- Heart block
- Tinnitus, fever
- Nausea, vomiting, diarrhea

Nursing Considerations
- Used for atrial or ventricular arrhythmias
- May increase toxicity for digitalis
- Monitor liver function tests and I and 0
- Check apical pulse and BP
- Monitor EKG and BP
- Avoid changing positions (lying/sitting/standing) rapidly
- Avoid use with alcohol, caffeine
- Patient should wear medical information tag
- Rx; Preg Cat C

• •

Side Effects
- Drowsiness, sedation
- Dry mouth
- Dizziness
- Headache
- Severe rebound hypertension

Nursing Considerations
- Treatment of hypertension, severe cancer pain (in combination with opiates)
- Avoid changing positions (lying/sitting/standing) rapidly
- Avoid use with alcohol, CNS depressants
- Avoid high sodium foods (canned soups, lunch meats, cheese)
- Use caution in potentially hazardous activities
- Avoid alcohol, smoking, strenuous exercise in hot environment
- Apply patch to non-hairy area (upper outer arm, anterior chest), rotate sites, do not apply to scarred or irritated area
- Wear medical identification tag
- Rx; Preg Cat C

HYDRALAZINE HCL
(hye-<u>dral</u>-a-zeen)
(Apresoline)

• •

HYDROCHLOROTHIAZIDE/LISINOPRIL
(hye-droe-klor-oh-<u>thye</u>-a-zide)
(Prinizide, Zestoretic)

Side Effects
  Headache
  Palpitations, tachycardia, angina
  Edema
  Lupus erythematosus-like syndrome
  Nausea, vomiting, diarrhea
  Anorexia
  Tremors
  Dizziness
  Anxiety

Nursing Considerations
  Used to treat essential hypertension
  PO: give with meals to enhance absorption
  Observe mental status
  Check for weight gain, edema
  Avoid changing positions (lying/sitting/standing) rapidly
  Contact clinician if chest pain, severe fatigue, fever, muscle or joint pain
  Rx; Preg Cat C

• •

Side Effects
  Headache
  Dizziness
  Hypotension
  Tachycardia
  Nausea, vomiting, diarrhea
  Fatigue

Nursing Considerations
  Used to treat essential hypertension
  Avoid changing positions (lying/sitting/standing) rapidly
  May take without regard to food
  Avoid high Na^+ foods (canned soups, lunch meats, cheese)
  Avoid high K^+ foods (bananas, citrus fruits, raisins)
  Rx; Preg Cat D

MINOXIDIL
(mi-<u>nox</u>-i-dill)
(Loniten, (Rogaine as topical treatment for hair loss))

• •

ATORVASTATIN CALCIUM
(at-ore-vuh-stat-in)
(Lipitor)

Side Effects
Edema
Increase in body hair

Nursing Considerations
Limited to treat severe symptomatic hypertension or uncontrolled by other means
Teach patient to take radial pulse
Check for weight gain, edema
Topical application (Rogaine) approved to promote hair growth in men and women
Rx; Preg Cat C

• •

Side Effects
Constipation
Abdominal pain
Nausea
Decreased vitamin A, D, K

Nursing Considerations
Used to lower cholesterol levels, digitalis toxicity, biliary obstruction pruritus, and diarrhea
Take other meds 1 hour before or 4 hours after this med to avoid poor absorption
Mix granules in applesauce or liquid, do not take dry, let stand for 2 minutes
Monitor for hypoprothrombinemia: bleeding gums, tarry stools, hematuria, bruising
Rx; Preg Cat B

COLESTIPOL
(koe-<u>les</u>-ti-pole)
(Colestid)

· ·

GEMFIBROZIL
(jem-<u>fi</u>-broe-zil)
(Lopid)

Side Effects
  Constipation
  Abdominal pain
  Nausea
  Decreased vitamin A, D, K

Nursing Considerations
  Used to lower choles-
  terol levels, digitalis toxicity,
  biliary obstruction pruritus,
  and diarrhea
  Take other meds 1 hour
  before or 4 hours after this
  med to avoid poor absorption
  Mix granules in applesauce
  or liquid, do not take dry, let
  stand for 2 minutes
  Monitor for hypoprothrombinemia: bleeding gums,
  tarry stools, hematuria,
  bruising
  Rx; Preg Cat B

• •

Side Effects
  Abdominal pain, diarrhea
  GI upset

Nursing Considerations
  Used to lower cholesterol
  levels
  Take 1/2 hour before meals
  Check CBC and liver func-
  tion tests
  PO: take 30 minutes before
  morning and evening meals
  May stop if no improvement
  in 3 months
  Rx; Preg Cat C

LOVASTATIN
(loh-vah-<u>stat</u>-in)
(Mevacor)

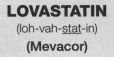

NIACIN
(<u>nye</u>-a-sin)
**(Niacor for immediate release;
Niaspan for sustained release)**

Side Effects

Flatus, constipation
Abdominal pain, nausea,
diarrhea, GI upset
Heartburn
Muscle cramps
Dizziness
Headache
Tremor
Blurred vision
Rash, pruritus

Nursing Considerations

Used to lower cholesterol
levels, primary and secondary
prevention of coronary events
Use sunscreen to prevent
photosensitivity reactions
Schedule liver function tests
every 1–2 months during
the first 1 1/2 years
Onset 2 weeks, peak 4–6
weeks, duration 6 weeks
Take with food, absorption
is reduced by 30 percent on
an empty stomach
Contact clinician if un-
explained muscle pain,
tenderness or weakness, esp.
if with fever or malaise
Rx; Preg Cat X

• •

Side Effects

Headache
Nausea
Postural hypotension

Nursing Considerations

Treatment of pellagra,
hyperlipidemias, peripheral
vascular disease
Take with meals to reduce
GI upset, can add 325 mg
ASA 1/2 hour before dose to
reduce flushing
Flushing will occur several
hours after med taken, will
decrease over 2 weeks
Avoid changing positions
(sitting/standing/lying)
rapidly
Rx/OTC; Preg Cat C

NICOTINIC ACID
(nih-koh-<u>tin</u>-ick)
(Slo-Niacin, Vitamin B)

· ·

PRAVASTATIN
(<u>pra</u>-va-sta-tin)
(Pravachol)

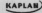

Side Effects
  Headache
  Nausea
  Postural hypotension

Nursing Considerations
  Treatment of pellagra,
  hyperlipidemias, peripheral
  vascular disease
  Take with meals to reduce
  GI upset, can add 325 mg
  ASA 1/2 hour before dose to
  reduce flushing
  Flushing will occur several
  hours after med taken, will
  decrease over 2 weeks
  Avoid changing positions
  (sitting/standing/lying)
  rapidly
  Rx/OTC; Preg Cat C

• •

Side Effects
  Abdominal cramps, flatus
  Constipation, diarrhea
  Heartburn

Nursing Considerations
  Treatment of hypercholes-
  terolemia, apolipoprotein B
  (apo B), risk reduction of re-
  current MI, atherosclerosis
  Schedule liver function tests
  semiannually
  Take without regard to food
  Contact clinician if
  unexplained muscle pain,
  tenderness or weakness,
  especially if with fever or
  malaise
  Rx; Preg Cat X

ROSUVASTATIN CALCIUM
(roe-sue-vuh-<u>stat</u>-in)
(Crestor)

· ·

SIMVASTATIN
(sim-va-<u>sta</u>-tin)
(Zocor)

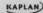

Side Effects
  Myalgia
  Constipation
  Abdominal pain
  Nausea

Nursing Considerations
  Used as adjunct therapy to
  diet to reduce LDL-C and
  increase HDL-C
  Patients should discontinue
  therapy and notify physician
  in case of pregnancy
  Use with caution in patients
  with a history of significant
  alcohol consumption
  Liver function tests are recommended every 12 weeks
  Patient should keep tight
  control of diet during
  therapy
  Rx; Preg Cat X

• •

Side Effects
  Eye lens opacities
  Liver dysfunction

Nursing Considerations
  Treatment of hypercho-
  lesterolemia, hypertriglyc-
  eridemia, hyperlipopro-
  teinemias, coronary artery
  disease
  Have eye exam before,
  1 month after, and then
  annually after starting med,
  lens opacities may occur
  Schedule liver function tests
  semiannually
  Take without regard to food
  Contact clinician if unexplained muscle pain, tenderness or weakness, especially
  if with fever or malaise
  Rx; Preg Cat X

ATENOLOL
(a-<u>ten</u>-oh-lole)
**(Tenormin, Tenoretic is combination
with Chlorthalidone)**

• •

CARVEDILOL
(kar-<u>ved</u>-i-lole)
(Coreg)

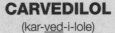

Side Effects	**Nursing Considerations**
Bradycardia, cold extremities	Used in treatment of hypertension, MI (IV use), prophylaxis of angina
Postural hypotension	Masks signs of hypoglycemia in diabetics
Bronchospasm in overdose	Teach patient how to take radial pulse
2nd or 3rd degree heart block	Check pulse, if less than 50 beats per minute, hold the med and contact clinician
Cold extremities	PO: Take before meals, at bedtime
Insomnia, fatigue	Tablet may be crushed or swallowed whole
Dizziness	Do not stop abruptly; taper over 2 weeks
Mental changes	Rx; Preg Cat D
Nausea, diarrhea	

• •

Side Effects	**Nursing Considerations**
Dizziness	Used in treatment of hypertension, CHF
Diarrhea	PO: Take with food
Postural hypotension	Tablet may be crushed or swallowed whole
Impotence	Do not stop abruptly; taper over 1–2 weeks
Hyperglycemia	Rx; Preg Cat C

METOPROLOL SUCCINATE, METOPROLOL TARTRATE
(meh-<u>toe</u>-proe-lole)
(ToprolXL, the sustained release form, Lopressor, the immediate release form)

· ·

PROPRANOLOL HCL
(proe-<u>pran</u>-oh-lole)
(Inderal)

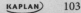

Side Effects
Bradycardia, palpitations
Hypotension
Congestive heart failure
Depression
Insomnia
Dizziness
Nausea, vomiting, diarrhea

Nursing Considerations
Used in treatment of
hypertension, MI (IV use),
prophylaxis of angina
Teach patient how to take
radial pulse
Check pulse, if less than 50
beats per minute, hold the
med and contact clinician
Do not stop abruptly; taper
over 2 weeks; may precipitate angina
Do not use OTC prod-
ucts (nasal decongestants,
cold preparations) unless
directed by prescriber
Rx; Preg Cat C

• •

Side Effects
Weakness
Hypotension
Bronchospasm
Bradycardia
Depression

Nursing Considerations
Used in treatment of
stable angina, hypertension,
dysrhythmias, migraine,
prophylaxis MI, essential
tremor, alcohol withdrawal
Teach patient how to take
radial pulse
Check pulse, if less than 50
beats per minute, hold the
med and contact clinician
PO: Take with full glass of

water at the same time each
day
Do not open, chew, crush
extended release capsule
Do not stop abruptly;
taper over 2 weeks; may
precipitate life-threatening
dysrhythmias
Do not use aluminum-
containing antacid; may
decrease absorption
Rx; Preg Cat C

AMLODIPINE BESYLATE
(am-<u>loh</u>-dip-ene)
(Norvasc)

• •

DILTIAZEM HCL
(dil-<u>tye</u>-a-zem)
**(Cardizem, Dilacor, Tiamate, Tiazac, Cardizem SR
(twice a day), Cardizem CD (once a day))**

Side Effects
Flushing
Edema
Headache
Fatigue

Nursing Considerations
Used to treat hypertension
Used also to treat vasospastic angina pectoris
May be taken without regards to meals
Consult physician before taking nonprescription cough remedies
Rx; Preg Cat C

Side Effects
Hypotension, dizziness
Edema
Nausea, constipation
Rash
Headache
Fatigue, drowsiness

Nursing Considerations
Management of angina, hypertension, vasospasm, atrial fibrillation, flutter, paroxysmal supraventricular tachycardia
Reduces workload of left ventricle, coronary vasodilator
Monitor blood pressure during dosage adjustments
PO: Take on an empty stomach, with a full glass of water
Teach patient how to take radial pulse and keep records of pulse rate
Avoid hazardous activities until stabilized on drug
Rx; Preg Cat C

NIFEDIPINE
(nye-<u>fed</u>-i-peen)
(Adalat CC, Procardia XL)

• •

VERAPAMIL HCL
(ver-<u>ap</u>-a-mill)
(Calan, Isoptin, Covera)

Side Effects

Orthostatic hypotension

Nursing Considerations

Used in treatment of hypertension, angina

Avoid changing positions (sitting/standing/lying) rapidly

PO: Take on an empty stomach; onset 20 minutes, peak 1/2–6 hours, duration 6–8 hours

PO of extended release capsule: do not open, chew, crush; can take without regard to meals; duration of 24 hours, shell may appear in stools, but is insignificant

Do not use OTC products or alcohol unless directed by prescriber; limit caffeine

Rx; Preg Cat C

• •

Side Effects

Edema

Nausea, constipation

Headache

Drowsiness

Nursing Considerations

Management of chronic stable angina, sysrhythmias, hypertension, supraventricular tachycardia, atrial flutter or fibrillation

PO: Take before meals, except sustained release to be taken with food

Do not open, chew, crush sustained or extended release capsule

Increased hypotensive effects with grapefruit juice

Teach patient how to take radial pulse and keep records of pulse rate

Avoid hazardous activities until stabilized on drug

Do not use OTC products or alcohol unless directed by prescriber; limit caffeine

Rx; Preg Cat C

DIGOXIN
(di-<u>jox</u>-in)
(Lanoxin)

. . . .

Cardiovascular Medications
LOOP DIURETICS

BUMETANIDE
(byoo-<u>met</u>-a-nide)
(Bumex)

Side Effects
Headache
Hypotension

Nursing Considerations
Used in treatment of CHF, atrial fibrillation, flutter or tachycardia, cardiogenic shock
Check pulse, if less than 60 beats per minute (adult) or 90 beats per minute (infant), hold the med and contact clinician
PO: with or without food; may crush tablets and mix with food/fluids
Do not open, chew, crush capsule

Contact clinician if loss of appetite, lower stomach pain, diarrhea, weakness, drowsiness, headache, blurred or yellow vision, rash, depression
Eat a sodium-restricted and potassium-rich (bananas, orange juice) diet to keep potassium level normal
Avoid OTC meds and herbals, many adverse interactions may occur
Rx; Preg Cat C

• •

Side Effects
Potassium depletion
Electrolyte imbalance
Hypovolemia
Ototoxicity
Hyperglycemia

Nursing Considerations
Used in treatment of hypertension
PO: diuresis onset 30–60 minutes, peak 1–2 hours, duration 3–6 hours
IM: diuresis onset 40 minutes, peak 1–2 hours, duration 4–6 hours
IV: diuresis onset 5 minutes, peak 15–30 minutes, duration 3–6 hours

Weigh daily
Do not take at bedtime to prevent nocturia
Encourage potassium-containing foods
Rx; Preg Cat C

FUROSEMIDE
(fur-<u>oh</u>-se-mide)
(Lasix)

. . . .

Cardiovascular Medications
PLATELET AGGREGATION INHIBITORS

CLOPIDOGREL BISULFATE
(klo-<u>pid</u>-oh-grel)
(Plavix)

Side Effects
Hypotension
Hypokalemia
Hyperglycemia
Nausea
Polyuria
Rash, pruritus

Nursing Considerations
Used in treatment of pulmonary edema, and edema in other conditions
PO: diuresis onset 60 minutes, peak 1–2 hours, duration 6–8 hours
IV: diuresis onset 5 minutes, peak 1/2 hour, duration 2 hours
PO: take with food or milk to prevent GI upset, slightly lessened absorption, tablets may be crushed
Take early in the day to prevent nocturia and sleeplessness
Avoid changing positions (sitting/standing/lying) rapidly
Use sunscreen or protective clothing to prevent photosensitivity
Rx; Preg Cat C

• •

Side Effects
GI bleeding
Nausea, vomiting, diarrhea, GI discomfort
Depression

Nursing Considerations
Used to reduce risk of stroke, MI, peripheral artery disease in high risk patients
Monitor blood studies in long-term therapy
Take with meals or just after to decrease gastric symptoms
Report signs of unusual bruising, bleeding; it may take longer to stop bleeding
Rx, Preg Cat B

DIPYRIDAMOLE
(dye-peer-<u>id</u>-a-mole)
(Persantine)

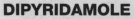

TICLOPIDINE HCL
(ty-<u>cloe</u>-pi-deen)
(Ticlid)

Side Effects
  Headache
  Dizziness
  Nausea, vomiting
  Postural hypotension
  Weakness, fainting, syncope
  Rash

Nursing Considerations
  Prevention of transient
  ischemic attacks, MIs, with
  warfarin in heart valves,
  with ASA in bypass grafts
  PO: peak in 2–2 1/2 hours;
  duration 6 hours
  PO: on an empty stomach,
  1 hour before or 2 hours
  after meals with full glass
  of water

  Full therapeutic response
  may take several months
  IV: do not give undiluted,
  give over 4 minutes
  Use caution with hazardous
  activities until stabilized on
  med
  Avoid changing positions
  (sitting/standing/lying)
  rapidly
  Rx; Preg Cat B

• •

Side Effects
  Rash
  Diarrhea
  Bleeding

Nursing Considerations
  Prevention of stroke in
  high-risk patients
  Monitor blood studies in
  long-term therapy
  Take with meals or just after
  to decrease gastric symptoms
  Monitor for signs of
  cholestasis (jaundice, dark
  urine, light-colored stools)
  Rx; Preg Cat B

HYDROCHLOROTHIAZIDE/
TRIAMTERENE

(hye-droe-klor-oh-<u>thye</u>-a-zide/trye-<u>am</u>-ter-een)

(Dyazide, Maxide)

· ·

SPIRONOLACTONE

(speer-in-oh-<u>lak</u>-tone)

(Aldactone)

Side Effects
Nausea, vomiting, diarrhea
Anemia

Nursing Considerations
Used in treatment of edema
and hypertension
Diuresis onset 2 hours
Take with meals or just after
to decrease gastric symp-
toms
Take early in the day to
prevent nocturia and sleeplessness
Rx; Preg Cat B

· ·

Side Effects
Hyperkalemia
Hyponatremia
Vomiting, diarrhea
Bleeding
Rash, pruritus

Nursing Considerations
Used in treatment of edema
and hypertension
Diuresis onset 24–48 hours,
peak 48–72 hours
Take in morning to avoid
interference with sleep
Take with meals or just after
to decrease gastric symp-
toms
Avoid food high in potas-
sium: oranges, bananas, salt

substitutes, dried apricots,
dates
Weigh daily to determine
fluid loss; effect of drug may
be decreased if used daily
Contact clinician if cramps,
lethargy, menstrual abnormalities, deepening voice,
breast enlargement
Rx; Preg Cat D

CHLORTHALIDONE
(klor-<u>thal</u>-i-done)
**(Hygroton, Hylidone, Thalitone;
Tenoretic is combination with ATENOLOL)**

. . . .

HYDROCHLOROTHIAZIDE
(hye-droe-klor-oh-<u>thye</u>-a-zide)
(Hydrodiuril)

Side Effects
- Dizziness
- Aplastic anemia
- Orthostatic hypotension
- Urinary frequency
- Fatigue, weakness
- Nausea, vomiting, anorexia
- Electrolyte changes

Nursing Considerations
Used in treatment of edema and hypertension
Diuresis onset 2 hours, peak 6 hours, duration 24–72 hours
Take with meals or just after to decrease gastric symptoms
Blood sugar may increase in diabetics
Take in morning to avoid interference with sleep
Weigh daily to determine fluid loss; effect of drug may be decreased if used daily
Avoid changing positions (sitting/standing/lying) rapidly
Rx; Preg Cat B

· ·

Side Effects
- Hypokalemia
- Hyperglycemia
- Blurred vision
- Fatigue, weakness
- Confusion, especially in elderly
- Nausea, vomiting, anorexia

Nursing Considerations
Used in treatment of edema and hypertension
Diuresis onset 2 hours, peak 4 hours, duration 6–12 hours
Take with meals or just after to decrease gastric symptoms
Blood sugar may increase in diabetics
Take in morning to avoid interference with sleep
Use sunscreen to prevent photosensitivity
Monitor for signs of hypokalemia: postural hypotension, malaise, fatigue, tachycardia, leg cramps, weakness, dehydration
Rx; Preg Cat B

INDAPAMIDE
(in-<u>dap</u>-a-mide)
(Lozol)

· ·

METOLAZONE
(me-<u>tole</u>-a-zone)
**(Diulo, Mykrox—prompt products,
Zaroxolyn—extended product)**

Side Effects
Headache
Electrolyte changes
Nausea
Rash, pruritus
Orthostatic hypotension

Nursing Considerations
Used in treatment of edema
of CHF and hypertension
Diuresis onset 1–2 hours,
peak 2 hours, duration
36 hours
Take with meals or just after
to decrease gastric symp-
toms, slightly decreased
absorption
Avoid changing positions
(sitting/standing/lying)
rapidly
Take in morning to avoid
interference with sleep
Monitor for signs of hypokalemia: postural hypo-
tension, malaise, fatigue,
tachycardia, leg cramps,
weakness, dehydration
Rx; Preg Cat B

• •

Side Effects
Dizziness, weakness, fatigue
Nausea, vomiting, anorexia
Rash
Hyperglycemia
Hypokalemia

Nursing Considerations
Used in treatment of edema
of CHF and hypertension
Diuresis onset 1 hour, peak
2 hours, duration 12–24
hours
Take with meals or just after
to decrease gastric symp-
toms, slightly decreased
absorption
Avoid changing positions
(sitting/standing/lying)
rapidly
Take in morning to avoid
interference with sleep
Use sunscreen to prevent
photosensitivity
Monitor for signs of hypokalemia: postural hypo-
tension, malaise, fatigue,
tachycardia, leg cramps,
weakness, dehydration
Rx; Preg Cat B

ISOTRETINOIN
(eye-sew-<u>treti</u>-noyn)
(Accutane)

• •

KETOCONAZOLE
(key-toe-<u>koe</u>-na-zol)
(Nizoral)

Side Effects
- Chilitis
- Conjunctivitis
- Dry skin
- Dry mouth
- Hair thinning

Nursing Considerations
Used to treat severe recalci-
trant cystic acne that does
not respond to conventional
therapy
Women of child bearing age
must have a negative pregnancy test for each month of
treatment
Rx; Preg Cat X

• •

Side Effects
- Dizziness
- Photophobia

Nursing Considerations
Treatment of fungal infections
C & S before first dose
PO: taken early A.M. with
food
Also available as a topical
cream or shampoo
Cannot take within two
hours of alkaline substances,
requires acid media to dissolve, follow with glass of
water
Take at the same time each
day

To prevent photophobia
in bright sunlight, wear
sunglasses
May require several weeks/
months of therapy
Avoid use of alcohol
Rx; Preg Cat C

NYSTATIN
(nye-<u>stat</u>-in)
(Mycostatin)

• •

Dermatologicals
ANTI-INFLAMMATORIES, TOPICAL

FLUCINONIDE
(floo-oh-<u>sin</u>-oh-lone)
(Lidex)

Side Effects

GI distress, hypersensitivity

Nursing Considerations

Treatment of Candida infections

Discontinue if redness, swelling, irritation occurs

Encourage good oral, vaginal, skin hygiene

Rx; Preg Cat C

- -

Side Effects

Acne
Atrophy
Epidermal thinning
Purpura
Striae

Nursing Considerations

Topical glucorticoid used to treat severe dermatoses not responding to less potent meds: psoriasis, eczema, contact dermatitis, pruritus

Apply only to affected areas; do not get in eyes

Leave site uncovered or lightly covered

Occlusive dressing is not recommended, systemic absorption may occur

Do not use on weeping, denuded, or infected areas

Avoid sunlight on affected area

Rx; Preg Cat C

TRIAMCINOLONE ACETONIDE
(trye-am-<u>sin</u>-oh-lone)
(Aristacort, Kenalog)

• •

Diabetic Medications
HYPOGLYCEMIC AGENTS, ORAL

GLIPIZIDE
(<u>glip</u>-i-zide)
(Glucotrol)

Side Effects
  Acne
  Atrophy
  Epidermal thinning
  Purpura
  Striae

Nursing Considerations
  Topical glucorticoid used to treat severe dermatoses not responding to less potent meds: psoriasis, eczema, contact dermatitis, pruritus
  Apply only to affected areas; do not get in eyes
  Leave site uncovered or lightly covered
  Occlusive dressing is not recommended, systemic absorption may occur
  Do not use on weeping, denuded, or infected areas
  Avoid sunlight on affected area
  Rx; Preg Cat C

• •

Side Effects
  Headache
  Weakness, dizziness
  Drowsiness

Nursing Considerations
  Management of stable adult-onset diabetes
  Do not drink alcohol since it can produce a disulfiram reaction: nausea, headache, cramps, flushing, hypoglycemia
  Assess for symptoms of cholestatic jaundice: dark urine, pruritus, yellow sclera (rare)
  XL: take at breakfast; onset is in 1–1 1/2 hours, peak in 1–3 hours, duration 10–24 hours
  Immediate release: take 30 minutes before meals, since absorption is delayed by food
  Have a quick source of sugar or a glucagon emergency kit available
  Use sun screen or protective clothing to prevent photo-sensitivity
  Extended release tablet coating may appear in stool
  Wear medical identification tag
  Rx; Preg Cat C

GLYBURIDE
(<u>glye</u>-byoo-ride)
(DiaBeta, Micronase)

. . . .

METFORMIN HCL
(met-<u>for</u>-min)
(Glucophage)

Side Effects
  Headache
  Weakness, dizziness

Nursing Considerations
  Management of stable adult-onset diabetes
  Assess for symptoms of cholestatic jaundice: dark urine, pruritus, yellow sclera (rare)
  Take at breakfast; onset is in 2–4 hours, peak in 4 hours, duration 24 hours
  Have a quick source of sugar or a glucagon emergency kit available
  Use sunscreen or protective clothing to prevent photo-sensitivity
  Wear medical identification tag
  Rx; Preg Cat B

● ●

Side Effects
  Headache
  Weakness, dizziness, drowsiness
  Agitation
  Nausea, vomiting, diarrhea
  Lactic acidosis

Nursing Considerations
  Management of stable adult-onset diabetes
  PO: twice a day with meals to decrease GI upset and provide best absorption; may also be taken as one dose
  Can crush tablets and mix with juice or soft foods for ease of swallowing

Do not crush, chew, or break extended release tablet; its coating may appear in stool
Be aware of signs of lactic acidosis: hyperventilation, fatigue, malaise, chills, myalgia, sleepiness
Have a quick source of sugar or a glucagon emergency kit available
Wear medical identification tag
Rx; Preg Cat B

REPAGLINIDE
(ree-<u>pag</u>-lihn-ide)
(Prandin)

· ·

ROSIGLITAZONE MALEATE
(row-se-<u>glit</u>-is-own)
(Avandia)

Side Effects
- Hyperglycemia
- Respiratory infection
- Headache
- Diarrhea
- Sinusitis

Nursing Considerations
Used to lower blood glucose levels in type 2 diabetes
Used in conjunction with diet and exercise regimen
Some antifungals may inhibit metabolism
Medication should be taken immediately before a meal
Dose should be skipped if meal is skipped
Rx; Preg Cat C

• •

Side Effects
- Upper respiratory infection
- Headache
- Back pain
- Hyperglycemia
- Fatigue

Nursing Considerations
Used in conjunction with diet and exercise to control blood glucose levels in patients with type 2 diabetes
Seldom used in type 1 diabetes because of the need for insulin to be present
May be taken at any time of day without regard to meals
Patient should be aware that rosiglitazone improves insulin sensitivity
Liver enzyme monitoring is recommended because of hepatotoxicity possibility
Rx; Preg Cat C

INSULIN ASPART
(Novolog)

• •

INSULIN GLARGINE
(Lantus)

Side Effects
Hypoglycemia
Lipodystrophy

Nursing Considerations
Management of diabetes
in adults. The only insulin
analog approved for use in
external pump systems for
continuous subQ insulin
infusion.
Onset 15 minutes, peak 1–3
hours, duration 3–5 hours
Never administer IV
Immediately follow injec-
tion with meal within 5–10
minutes
Rx; Preg Cat B

• •

Side Effects
Hypoglycemia
Lipodystrophy

Nursing Considerations
Management of diabetes in
type 1 diabetics or adults
with type 2 requiring a long-
acting insulin to control
hyperglycemia
Onset 1.1 hours, peak 5
hours, duration 24 hours
Not the drug of choice for
diabetic ketoacidosis (use a
short-acting insulin)
Higher incidence of injection site pain compared
with NPH
Rx; Preg Cat C

INSULIN, ISOPHANE SUSPENSION (NPH)
(Humulin N, Novolin N)

• •

INSULIN LISPRO
(Humalog)

Side Effects
Hypoglycemia
Lipodystrophy

Nursing Considerations
Management of diabetes
Comes in 100 units per
milliliter vial as well as in
combination with regular
insulin in a 50/50 proportion and a 70/30 proportion
subQ: onset 1–1 1/2 hours,
peak 4–12 hours, duration
18–24 hours
Rx; Preg Cat B

• •

Side Effects
Hypoglycemia
Lipodystrophy

Nursing Considerations
Management of type 1
diabetes and in combination
with sulfonylureas for type
2 diabetes
Take within 15 minutes of
eating and immediately
after mixing, with combined
therapy
May be used in children in
combination with sulfonylureas
Onset rapid, peak 1/2–1 1/2
hour, duration 6–8 hours
Rx; Preg Cat B

INSULIN, REGULAR
(Novolin R)

. . . .

INSULIN, REGULAR CONCENTRATED
(Iletin II U-500)

Side Effects
  Hypoglycemia
  Lipodystrophy

Nursing Considerations
  Management of diabetic
  coma, diabetic acidosis, or
  other emergency conditions.
  Especially suitable for labile
  diabetes. Used in external
  insulin infusion pumps
  Comes in 100 units per milliliter vial
  Only insulin that can be
  given IV
  subQ: onset 1/2–1 hour,
  peak 10–30 minutes, duration 1/2–1 hour
  IV: onset 10–30 minutes,
  peak 10–30 minutes, duration 1/2–1 hour
  Rx; Preg Cat B

• •

Side Effects
  Hypoglycemia
  Lipodystrophy

Nursing Considerations
  Management of insulin-
  resistant diabetes requiring
  more than 200 units insulin
  per day
  Comes in 500 units per milliliter vial
  subQ: onset 1/2–1 hour,
  peak 2–5 hours, duration
  5–7 hours
  Deep secondary hypogly-
  cemia 18–24 hours after
  injection; monitor closely
  and have 10–20% dextrose
  solution available
  Record blood sugar 2 hours
  post-prandial
  Rx; Preg Cat B

INSULIN, ZINC SUSPENSION (LENTE)
(Humulin L, Novolin L)

• •

INSULIN, ZINC SUSPENSION
EXTENDED (ULTRALENTE)
(Humulin U Ultralente, Novolin U, Ultralente U)

Side Effects
  Hypoglycemia
  Lipodystrophy

Nursing Considerations
  Management of diabetes
  in patients allergic to other
  types of insulin and those
  disposed to thrombotic phe-
  nomena in which protamine
  may be a factor
  Comes in 100 units per
  milliliter vial
  subQ: Onset 1–2 1/2 hours,
  peak 7–15 hours, duration
  18–24 hours
  Not a replacement for
  regular insulin and is not
  suitable for emergency use
  Rx; Preg Cat B

• •

Side Effects
  Hypoglycemia
  Lipodystrophy

Nursing Considerations
  Management of mild to
  moderate hyperglycemia in
  stabilized diabetics
  Comes in 100 units per
  milliliter vial
  Large crystals of insulin and
  a high content of size are
  responsible for the slow-act-
  ing properties
  subQ: onset 4–8 hours, peak
  10–30 hours, duration
  36 hours or longer
  Rx; Preg Cat B

GLUCAGON
(<u>gloo</u>-ka-gon)
(GlucaGen)

* *

Gastrointestinal Medications
ANTACIDS

ALUMINUM HYDROXIDE GEL
(Amphojel)

Side Effects
Nausea, vomiting

Nursing Considerations
Acute management of severe hypoglycemia; facilitation of GI x-rays
IM for hypoglycemia: onset within 10 minutes, peak 30 minutes, duration 60–90 minutes
IV for hypoglycemia: onset within 10 minutes, peak 5 minutes, duration 60–90 minutes
SubQ for hypoglycemia: onset within 10 minutes, peak 30–45 minutes, duration 60–90 minutes

IV for GI x-rays: onset within 45 seconds, duration dose dependent of 9–25 minutes
IM for GI x-rays: onset within 8–10 minutes, duration dose dependent of 9–32 minutes
Rx/OTC; Preg Cat B

• •

Side Effects
Constipation that may lead to impaction
Phosphate depletion

Nursing Considerations
Antacid with duration of effect of 20 to 180 minutes
Aluminum antacid compounds interfere with tetracycline absorption
Contact clinician if signs of GI bleeding: tarry stools or coffee-grounds vomitus
Shake suspension well and follow with small amount of milk or water to facilitate passage
Monitor long-term, high-dose use if on restricted sodium intake, due to high sodium content
If prolonged use, monitor for phosphate depletion: anorexia, malaise, and muscle weakness; can also lead to resorption of calcium and bone demineralization in uremia patients
Use may interfere with some imaging techniques
Because drug contains aluminum, used in renal failure to control hyperphosphatemia by binding with phosphate in the GI tract
OTC; Preg Cat B

ALUMINUM HYDROXIDE AND MAGNESIUM TRISILICATE
(Riopan)

· ·

CALCIUM CARBONATE
(Tums)

Side Effects
   Mild constipation
   Diarrhea
   Increased urine pH levels
   Hypophosphotemia

Nursing Considerations
   Antacid with onset in
   20 minutes and duration of
   20–180 minutes
   May decrease effect of
   antibiotics and other drugs,
   such as digoxin, phenothi-
   azines, quinidine, salicylates
   due to impaired absorption,
   so separate administration
   times by 1–2 hours
   Since low sodium content,
   used in patients on sodium
   restriction
   If given with enteric-coated
   drugs, might have premature release in stomach;
   separate administration
   times by at least 1 hour
   Shake suspension well and
   follow with small amount of
   water to facilitate passage
   Contact clinician if signs of
   GI bleeding: tarry stools or
   coffee-grounds vomitus
   OTC; Preg Cat B

• •

Side Effects
   Nausea

Nursing Considerations
   Used as antacid and calcium
   supplement
   May decrease effect of some
   antibiotics and other drugs
   due to impaired absorption,
   so separate administration
   times by 2 hours
   Do not use if ventricular
   fibrillation or hypercalcemia
   Use caution if taking cardiac
   glycoside or has sarcoidosis
   or renal or cardiac disease
   Signs of hypercalcemia:
   nausea, vomiting, headache,
   confusion, anorexia
   OTC; Preg Cat B

DICYCLOMINE HCL
(dye-<u>sye</u>-kloh-meen)
(Bentyl)

. . . .

HYOSCYAMINE
(hye-oh-<u>sye</u>-a-meen)
(Anaspaz, Gastrosed)

Side Effects	**Nursing Considerations**
Drowsiness	Used for treatment of
Blurred vision	irritable bowel syndrome
	Take 30 minutes before
	meals and at bedtime
	Use caution with potentially
	hazardous activities
	Rx; Preg Cat C

• •

Side Effects	**Nursing Considerations**
Confusion, stimulation in elderly	Treatment of peptic ulcer, other GI disorders, other
Dry mouth, constipation	spastic disorders, urinary
Urinary retention, hesitancy	incontinence
Palpitations	PO: onset 20–30 minutes,
Blurred vision	duration 4–6 hours
	IM, IV, subQ: onset
	2–3 minutes, duration
	4–6 hours
	Avoid activities requiring
	alertness until stabilized on
	med
	Avoid alcohol, other CNS
	depressants
	Use sunglasses to prevent
	photophobia
	Rx; Preg Cat C

LOPERAMIDE HCL
(loe-<u>per</u>-a-mide)
(Imodium)

• •

MECLIZINE
(<u>mek</u>-li-zeen)
(Antivert, Bonine)

Side Effects
 Nausea, vomiting
 Abdominal pain/distention
 Dizziness
 Drowsiness
 Dry mouth

Nursing Considerations
 Used for control of diarrhea, including diarrhea in
 travelers
 Take with a full glass of H_2O
 Encourage 6–8 glasses of
 fluid per day
 Use caution with potentially
 hazardous activities
 If abdominal distention in
 acute ulcerative colitis, stop
 med

 Avoid use with alcohol, CNS
 depressants
 Follow clear liquid or bland
 diet until diarrhea subsides
 Do not use OTC if fever
 over 101°F (38°C) or if
 bloody diarrhea
 Rx/OTC; Preg Cat B

• •

Side Effects
 Drowsiness
 Dizziness

Nursing Considerations
 Management of vertigo, mo-
 tion sickness
 Duration 8–14 hours
 Take 1 hour before traveling
 Avoid activities requiring
 alertness
 Avoid alcohol, other CNS
 depressants
 OTC/Rx; Preg Cat B

METOCLOPRAMIDE HCL
(met-oh-<u>kloe</u>-pra-mide)

(Reglan)

· ·

PROCHLORPERAZINE
(proe-klor-<u>pair</u>-a-zeen)

(Compazine)

Side Effects
  Drowsiness
  Restlessness
  Lassitude
  Headache
  Sleeplessness
  Dry mouth
  Anxiety

Nursing Considerations
  Prevention of nausea, vomiting induced by chemotherapy, radiation, delayed gastric emptying, GERD
  Used with tube feeding to decrease residual and risk of aspiration
  PO: Take 1/2 hour–1 hour before meals or procedures
  IV: Inject slowly over 1–2 minutes; infuse over 15 minutes
  Use caution with potentially hazardous activities
  Avoid alcohol and other CNS depressants
  Rx; Preg Cat B

• •

Side Effects
  Orthostatic hypotension
  Blurred vision
  Dry eyes, dry mouth
  Constipation
  Drowsiness
  Photosensitivity

Nursing Considerations
  Management of nausea, vomiting, psychotic disorders
  Monitor for development of neuroleptic malignant syndrome (fever, respiratory distress, tachycardia, convulsions, sweating, hypertension or hypotension, pallor, tiredness, severe muscle stiffness, loss of bladder control)

Notify clinician immediately
PO: Take with food
Do not crush or break sustained release capsules
IM: inject slowly, deeply into gluteal UOQ; keep patient lying down for 30 minutes
Use caution with potentially hazardous activities
Avoid changing positions (lying/sitting/standing) rapidly
Wear sunscreen and protective clothing to prevent photosensitivity reactions
Check CBC and liver functions with prolonged use
Rx; Preg Cat C

PROMETHAZINE
(pro-<u>meth</u>-a-zeen)
(Phenergan)

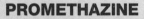

Gastrointestinal Medications
ANTIFLATULENTS

SIMETHICONE
(si-<u>meth</u>-i-kone)

Side Effects
Drowsiness
Dizziness
Constipation
Urinary retention
Dry mouth

Nursing Considerations
Management of motion
sickness, rhinitis, allergy
symptoms, sedation, nausea,
pre and post-operative
sedation
PO: onset 20 minutes, duration 4–6 hours
Take 1/2–1 hour before
traveling
Avoid activities requiring
alertness
Avoid alcohol, other CNS
depressants
Rx; Preg Cat C

• •

Side Effects
Belching
Rectal flatus

Nursing Considerations
Helps disperse gas pock-
ets in GI system, does not
decrease gas production
Take after meals, at bedtime
Shake suspension well
before pouring
Tablets must be chewed
Rx/OTC; Preg Cat C

ESOMEPRAZOLE MAGNESIUM

(e-sew-<u>mep</u>-ruh-zole)

(Nexium)

• •

OMEPRAZOLE

(oh-<u>meh</u>-pruh-zole)

(Prilosec)

Side Effects
  Headache
  Diarrhea
  Nausea
  Flatulence
  Dry mouth

Nursing Considerations
  Short term treatment of
  erosive esophagitis
  Used to treat gastroesopha-
  geal reflux disease (GERD)
  Take at least 60 minutes
  before meals
  Swallow capsules whole, do
  not chew
  May be taken in conjunc-
  tion with antacids
  Rx; Preg Cat B

• •

Side Effects
  Rare

Nursing Considerations
  Treatment of active duodenal
  ulcers
  Treatment of gastroesopha-
  geal reflux disease (GERD)
  in patients over 2
  Take 30 minutes before
  eating
  May be taken at the same
  time as antacids
  Rx/OTC: Preg Cat C

CIMETIDINE
(sye-<u>met</u>-ih-deen)

(Tagamet)

· ·

FAMOTIDINE
(fa-<u>moe</u>-ti-deen)

(Pepcid)

Side Effects
Diarrhea
Confusion (especially in elderly with large doses)
Headache
Dysrhythmias

Nursing Considerations
Reduces gastric acid secretions by 50–80%
May be taken without regard to meals
Avoid antacids 1 hour before or after dose
Do not use OTC for more than 2 weeks unless medically supervised
Monitor liver enzymes and blood counts
OTC/Rx; Preg Cat B

• •

Side Effects
Headache
Dizziness
Constipation
Blood dyscrasias

Nursing Considerations
Treatment of duodenal and gastric ulcers, gastro-esophageal reflux disease, heartburn
PO: onset 30–60 minutes, peak 1–3 hours, duration 6–12 hours
IV: onset immediate, peak 30–60 minutes, duration 8–15 hours
Signs of blood dyscrasia: bleeding, bruising, fatigue, malaise, poor healing
OTC/Rx; Preg Cat B

LANSOPRAZOLE
(lan-<u>so</u>-prey-zohl)
(Prevacid)

· ·

MISOPROSTOL
(mis-oh-<u>prost</u>-ole)
(Cytotec)

Side Effects
Dizziness
Diarrhea

Nursing Considerations
Used for treatment of GERD
and ulcers
PO: Take no more than
30 minutes before meals
Capsules may be opened
and sprinkled on food
(applesauce, pudding, cot-
tage cheese, yogurt) and
swallowed immediately
Can use with antacids
Do not crush or chew cap-
sule contents
To give with NG tube in
place, open the capsule and
mix with orange, apple or
tomato juice, instill through
NG tube and flush with ad-
ditional juice to clear tube
Report severe diarrhea
Rx; Preg Cat B

• •

Side Effects
Abdominal pain
Diarrhea (13%)
Miscarriage

Nursing Considerations
Prevention of gastric ulcers
during NSAIA therapy
Take with meals and at
bedtime
Avoid taking magnesium
antacids within 2 hours
Notify clinician if diarrhea
lasts more than 1 week
Notify clinician if black,
tarry stools or severe abdominal pain
Rx; Preg Cat X

RABEPRAZOLE
(rah-<u>bep</u>-rah-zole)
(Aciphex)

• •

RANITIDINE
(ra-<u>nit</u>-i-deen)
(Zantac)

Side Effects
   Headache
   Dizziness
   Nausea, vomiting, diarrhea
   Constipation, flatulence
   Rash
   Back pain

Nursing Considerations
   Used for treatment of GERD
   and duodenal ulcers
   Take on an empty stomach
   before eating
   Swallow tablets whole; do
   not crush, chew or split
   tablets
   Avoid alcohol, NSAIDs and
   ASA; may increase gastric
   upset
   Rx; Preg Cat B

• •

Side Effects
   Dizziness (especially in
   elderly)
   Drowsiness
   Headache

Nursing Considerations
   Used to inhibit gastric acid
   secretion
   Take with or immediately
   following meals
   Do not take antacids within
   1 hour before or after
   Do not smoke; it interferes
   with healing and drug's effectiveness
   Avoid alcohol, ASA, and
   caffeine which increase
   stomach acid
   Rx/OTC; Preg Cat B

SUCRALFATE
(soo-<u>kral</u>-fate)
(Carafate)

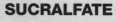

SULFASALAZINE
(sul-fah-<u>sal</u>-ah-zeen)
(Azulfidine)

Side Effects
   Constipation

Nursing Considerations
   Short-term treatment (less
   than 8 weeks) of duodenal
   ulcers
   PO: 1 hour before meals or
   2 hours after meals and at hs
   with full glass of water
   Do not chew tablets
   Do not use antacids within
   half an hour of med
   Encourage 8–10 glasses of
   fluid per day
   Avoid use with smoking
   Rx; Preg Cat B

• •

Side Effects
   Headache
   Anorexia
   Nausea, vomiting, diarrhea
   Rashes
   Fever

Nursing Considerations
   Used for treatment of inflammatory bowel diseases
   and arthritis
   PO: Take with food to
   decrease GI upset
   Encourage fluids to decrease
   crystalization in kidneys
   May permanently stain
   contact lens yellow
   May cause orange-yellow
   urine and skin, which is not
   significant
   Wear sunscreen and protective clothing to prevent
   photosensitivity reactions
   Rx; Preg Cat B

PHENTERMINE
(<u>fen</u>-ter-meen)
(Ionamin)

• •

SIBUTRAMINE
(sy-<u>bo</u>-truh-mine)
(Meridia)

Side Effects
  CNS stimulation
  Hypertension
  Palpitations
  Drowsiness

Nursing Considerations
  Short-term treatment of
  obesity
  PO: hydrochloride form
  duration is 4 hours
  PO: resin complex form
  duration is 12–14 hours
  Take 30 minutes before
  meals or as a single dose
  before breakfast or 10–14
  hours before bedtime
  Avoid activities requiring
  alertness until response is
  known
  Avoid alcohol, other CNS
  depressants
  Contact clinician if chest
  pain, decreased exercise
  tolerance, fainting or lower
  extremity swelling
  Rx; Schedule IV; Preg Cat C

• •

Side Effects
  Headache
  Dry mouth
  Anorexia
  Constipation
  Insomnia
  Rhinitis
  Back pain

Nursing Considerations
  Used to manage weight loss
  and maintenance in obesity
  Should be used with a
  reduced-calorie diet
  Regular heart rate and
  blood pressure monitoring
  is important
  Avoid use with Monoamine
  Oxidase Inhibitors
  Should not be used in pa-
  tients with cardiac disease
  Rx; Schedule C-IV; Preg
  Cat C

LACTULOSE SYRUP
(<u>lak</u>-tyoo-lose)
(Cephulac, Duphalac, Enulose)

• •

PANCREATIN
(<u>pan</u>-kree-a-tin)

Side Effects
Nausea, vomiting
Abdominal cramps

Nursing Considerations
Used for chronic
constipation
PO: Take with water or fruit
juice to counteract sweet
taste
Rx; Preg Cat B

● ●

Side Effects
Anorexia
Nausea, vomiting, diarrhea

Nursing Considerations
Do not crush or break
enteric-coated capsules
Do not use if sensitivity or
allergy to pork
Rx; Preg Cat C

PANCRELIPASE

(pan-kree-<u>ly</u>-payz)

(Pancrease, Viokase)

• •

Genitourinary Medications
ANTICHOLINERGICS

OXYBUTYNIN CHLORIDE

(ox-i-<u>byoo</u>-ti-nin)

(Ditropan)

Side Effects	Nursing Considerations
Abdominal pain (high doses only)	Used to replace or supplement naturally occurring enzymes, contains lipase, amylase, and protease
Nausea, diarrhea	
Stomach cramps	Take with 8 ounces of water and food, swallow right away, sit up when taking
	Do not crush or break enteric-coated capsules
	Do not use if sensitivity or allergy to pork
	Stools will be foul-smelling and frothy
	Rx; Preg Cat C

• •

Side Effects	Nursing Considerations
Anxiety, restlessness	Antispasmodic treatment of neurogenic bladder
Dizziness	
Convulsions	Take on an empty stomach
Palpitations, tachycardia	Avoid alcohol, other CNS depressants
Nausea, vomiting	
Anorexia	Avoid activities requiring alertness until med response is known
Drowsiness, blurred vision	
Dry mouth	Decreased ability to perspire means avoid strenuous activity in warm weather
Mydriasis	
	Wear sunglasses in bright sunlight to prevent photophobia
	Rx; Preg Cat B

TOLTERODINE TARTRATE
(toal-tear-oh-dene)
(Detrol, Detrol LA)

• •

SILDANAFIL CITRATE
(sil-<u>den</u>-a-fill)
(Viagra)

Side Effects
  Dry mouth
  Dizziness
  Constipation
  Dyspepsia
  Somnolence

Nursing Considerations
  Used to treat patients with overactive bladder
  Effective with frequency, urgency, or incontinence symptoms
  Patients should avoid alcohol during treatment with tolterodine
  Missed doses should be skipped, return to normal schedule
  Rx; Preg Cat C

• •

Side Effects
  Headache, flushing
  Dizziness
  Upset stomach
  Nasal congestion
  UTI
  Abnormal vision
  Rash

Nursing Considerations
  Treatment of erectile dysfunction
  Take approximately 1 hour before sexual activity
  Do not use more than once a day
  Tablets may be split
  High-fat meal will reduce absorption; better absorption on empty stomach
  Never use with nitrates; could have fatal fall in blood pressure
  Notify clinician if erection lasts longer than 4 hours
  Rx; Preg Cat B

TADALAFIL
(the-<u>dal</u>-uh-fil)
(Cialis)

• •

VARDENAFIL
(var-<u>den</u>-uh-fil)
(Levitra)

Side Effects
- Headache
- Dispepsia
- Back pain
- Flushing

Nursing Considerations
- Used to treat erectile dysfunction
- Patients with severe hepatic impairment should not take tadalafil
- Contraindicated in patients taking nitrates or alpha-adergenic blockers
- Tadalafil does not protect against sexually-transmitted diseases
- Alert physician if erection lasts more than four hours
- Rx; Preg Cat B

• •

Side Effects
- Headache
- Flushing
- Nasal congestion
- Dyspepsia

Nursing Considerations
- Used to treat erectile dysfunction
- Does not protect against sexually transmitted diseases
- Contraindicated in patients taking organic nitrates
- Contact physician if erection lasts over 4 hours
- Plasma levels peak in 30 minutes to 2 hours
- Rx; Preg Cat B

FINASTERIDE
(fin-<u>as</u>-the-ride)
(Proscar, Propecia)

• •

Genitourinary Medications
URINARY ANALGESICS

PHENAZOPYRIDINE HCL
(fen-az-oh-<u>peer</u>-i-deen)
(Azo, Pyridium)

Side Effects
  Decreased libido
  Impotence
  Breast tenderness
  Decreased volume of
  ejaculate

Nursing Considerations
  Treatment of benign prostatic hyperplasia (BPH) by
  Proscar, male hair loss by
  Propecia
  May be taken without
  regard for food
  Pregnant women should
  avoid contact with crushed
  drug or patient's semen;
  may adversely affect devel-
  oping male fetus
  Full therapeutic effect: Propecia may require 3 months,
  Proscar may require 6–12
  months
  Rx; Preg Cat X

• •

Side Effects
  GI upset
  Kidney and liver toxicity

Nursing Considerations
  Treatment of urinary tract
  irritation, often paired with
  urinary anti-infective
  Can crush tablets for ease of
  swallowing; can take with
  food or milk to decrease GI
  upset
  Inform patient that urine
  will be bright orange/red;
  may stain clothes or contact
  lens
  Monitor for signs of hepa-
  toxicity: dark urine, clay-
  colored stools, jaundice,
  itching, abdominal pain,
  fever, diarrhea
  Rx/OTC; Preg Cat B

NITROFURANTOIN
(nye-troe-<u>fyoor</u>-an-toyn)
(Furadantin, Macrobid, Macrodantin)

• •

Herbs/Botanicals

ALOE VERA
(al-oh-<u>vair</u>-ah)

Side Effects
Dizziness
Nausea, vomiting, diarrhea
Abdominal pain
Tooth staining

Nursing Considerations
Treatment of urinary tract infections
Take with food or milk
Avoid alcohol
Two daily doses if urine output is high or patient has diabetes
Drug may turn urine rust-yellow to brown
Rx; Preg Cat B

• •

Side Effects
Rare contact dermatitis

Nursing Implications
Wound healing and treatment of skin conditions such as burns and abrasions. Ingredient in hundreds of skin products, including lotions and sunblocks. Check label. Not for use on deep surgical wounds. Gel does not prevent burns from radiation therapy
If taken internally, abdominal cramping and diarrhea
Causes reduced absorption of other medications. Not recommended, especially for diabetics.

BLACK COHASH
(blak koe-hash)

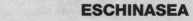

ESCHINASEA
(ess-kin-<u>ay</u>-jah)

Side Effects
Headaches
Stomach discomfort
Heaviness in legs
Weight problems

Nursing Implications
Used to treat menopausal symptoms, menstrual irregularities and PMS and to induce labor
No reported interactions with other medications
No long-term safety data available. No data supporting use by women who have breast cancer or are pregnant

• •

Side Effects
Heart palpitations, seizure, heart attack, stroke, death

Nursing Implications
Since not a prescribed medication, encourage users to report if they self-prescribe and use it
People with allergies to the daisy or sunflower family should avoid use
Might counteract immune-suppressant drugs such as glucocorticoids taken for lupus and rheumatoid arthritis. Might increase side effects of methotrexate.

FEVERFEW
(<u>fee</u>-ver-fyoo)

· ·

GARLIC
(<u>gar</u>-lick)

Side Effects	Nursing Implications
Canker sores	Used to treat migraine
Swelling and irritation of	headaches and rheumatoid
lips and tongue	arthritis
Loss of taste	If sudden discontinuation
Nausea, digestive problems,	after long-time use, head-
bloating	aches, nervousness, diffi-
	culty sleeping, stiff muscles,
	and joint pain
	Not for pregnant women
	since can cause uterine
	contractions
	People with allergies to
	the daisy family (including
	ragweed and mums) should
	avoid use

• •

Side Effects	Nursing Implications
Breath and body odor	Used to treat high choles-
Heartburn, upset stomach,	terol, heart disease, and high
allergic reactions	blood pressure
All side effects more com-	Can interfere with HIV
mon with raw garlic	drugs
	Use with caution if dental
	work or surgery as garlic
	thins blood like aspirin
	Avoid use for one week
	prior
	Avoid use if bleeding
	disorder
	Can increase effects of
	blood thinning drugs and
	other herbs

GINGER
(jin-jer)

· ·

GINKO BILOBA
(<u>gin</u>-koe bill-<u>oh</u>-bah)

Side Effects

Gas, bloating, heartburn, nausea

Side effects more common with powdered ginger

Nursing Implications

Used to treat stomach aches, nausea and diarrhea

Safe relief of pregnancy-related nausea and vomiting. Not proven in other situations, such as motion sickness, chemotherapy or post-surgery

Can increase NSAID side effects and effects of blood thinning drugs and other herbs

Ingredient in many digestive, antinausea and cold and flu dietary supplements

Check label

• •

Side Effects

Increased bleeding risk

Uncooked ginko seeds can cause seizures. Ingestion of large quantity over time can cause death

Headache

Nausea, GI upset, diarrhea

Dizziness

Allergic skin reactions

Nursing implications

Used to for memory enhancement, intermittent claudication, tinnitus

Due to bleeding risk increase, caution with anti-coagulant drugs, bleeding disorders, scheduled surgery or dental work

May increase circulation in Raynaud's Syndrome

Can increase effects of blood thinning drugs and other herbs

GINSENG
(<u>gin</u>-seng)

• •

GOLDENSEAL
(<u>goal</u>-den-seel)

Side Effects
Headaches
Sleep problems
GI difficulties

Nursing Implications
Research results have not
proven health claims
May lower blood glucose
Effect stronger in diabetics,
so caution urged
Possible beneficial effects on
immune function. Studies
being conducted on treat-
ing chronic lung infection,
impaired glucose tolerance,
and Alzheimer's disease
May increase effects of
blood-thinning drugs,
estrogens
May interact with MAO
inhibitors

• •

Side Effects
Nausea, vomiting

Nursing Implications
Ingredient often combined
with Echinacea in cold
remedies
Considered safe for adults,
but should not be given to
infants and young children
Other herbs are sometimes
substituted for goldenseal
with different effects
Pregnant and breast-feeding
women should avoid use
Premature labor or miscarriage could result. Life-
threatening liver problems
in nursing infants could
happen

KAVA
(<u>kah</u>-vah)

• •

SAW PALMETTO
(saw pahl-<u>met</u>-toe)

Side Effects

Liver damage, including hepatitis and possibly fatal liver failure (FDA warning issued)

Dystonia (abnormal muscle spasm or involuntary muscle movement)

Drowsiness

Scaly, yellowed skin with long-term or heavy use

Nursing Implications

Used to treat anxiety, insomnia and menopausal symptoms

Interaction with drugs used for Parkinson's disease

Avoid driving and using heaving machinery while using kava

Do not use with alcohol or antidepressants

Can increase effect of sedatives and tranquilizers

• •

Side Effects

Stomach discomfort

Tender breasts

Decline in sexual desire

Nursing Implications

Used to treat urinary symptoms of benign prostatic hypertrophy (BPH)

Does not affect PSA test readings to screen for possible prostate cancer and to monitor patients who have had prostate cancer

ST. JOHN'S WORT

• •

VALERIAN ROOT

Side Effects	Nursing Implications
Anxiety	Treatment of mild to moderate depression, anxiety, sleep disorders
Dry mouth	
Dizziness	
GI symptoms	Not for serious depression
Fatigue	Interaction with broad spectrum of medications, sometimes speeding drug breakdown, sometimes slowing it. Can interfere with many drugs' effectiveness, including meds for HIV, heart disease, transplant rejection, depression, anticoagulation, cancer, oral contraceptives
Headache	
Sexual dysfunction	
Photosensitivity	
	Can increase effect of alcohol and narcotics
	Can interfere with iron absorption

• •

Side Effects	Nursing Implications
Headaches	Used to treat insomnia
Dizziness	Considered generally safe for short-term (4–6 weeks) use
Upset stomach	
Tiredness the morning after its use	Do not use with alcohol or antidepressants
	Can increase effect of sedatives and tranquilizers
	No information about long-term safety

ALENDRONATE
(al-en-<u>drone</u>-ate)
(Fosamax)

• •

IBANDRONATE
(eye-<u>ban</u>-droh-nate)
(Boniva)

Side Effects
Esophageal ulceration

Nursing Considerations
Treatment of osteoporosis
in postmenopausal women
and in men, Paget's disease
Onset: 1 month, peak 3–6
months, duration 3 weeks to
7 months
Take in A.M. before food or
other meds with full glass of
water; remain upright for 30
minutes
If dose missed, skip dose,
do not double doses or take
later in the day
Take with calcium and
Vitamin D if instructed by
clinician
Rx; Preg Cat C

• •

Side Effects
Nausea, stomach pain, diar-
rhea, constipation
Bone, joint or muscle pain
Weakness, dizziness
Headache
Flu-like symptoms, fever,
sore throat, chills, cough,
and other signs of infection

Nursing Considerations
Treatment of osteoporosis,
Paget's disease, bone metastases. Will lower elevated
levels of blood calcium in
cancer patients
Contact prescriber if new
or worsening heartburn,
swallowing difficulty, or jaw
problems
Rx; Preg Cat C

RALOXIFENE
(rah-lox-ih-feen)
(Evista)

· ·

RISEDRONATE
(riss-<u>ed</u>-roe-nate)
(Actonel)

Side Effects

Hot flashes, more common
in first 6 months
Leg cramps
Swelling of extremities

Nursing Considerations

Prevention and treatment of
osteoporosis
Increases risk of blood clots.
Discuss prevention activities
Notify prescriber if sudden
chest pain or chest heaviness, difficulty breathing,
coughing up blood, swelling
or vision changes
Rx; Preg Cat X

• •

Side Effects

Weakness
Diarrhea, abdominal pain
Bone pain

Nursing Considerations

Treatment of osteoporosis
in postmenopausal women
and for Paget's disease
Onset: within days, peak
30 days, duration up to 16
months
Take in A.M. before food or
other meds with full glass of
water; remain upright for 30
minutes
Take with calcium and
Vitamin D if instructed by
clinician
Rx; Preg Cat C

ETIDRONATE
(eh-tih-<u>droe</u>-nate)
(Didronel)

• •

Hormones/Synthetic Substitutes/Modifiers
THYROID HORMONES

THYROID
(<u>thigh</u>-royd)
(Armour Thyroid)

Side Effects
Nausea, diarrhea
Bone pain and tenderness

Nursing Considerations
Treatment of Paget's disease, used with total hip replacement and spinal cord injury, hypercalemia of cancer
PO: onset 1 month, duration 1 year
IV: onset 24 hours, peak 3 days, duration 11 days
Take on empty stomach with calcium and Vitamin D but not within 2 hours of med
Contact clinician if sudden onset of unexpected pain, restricted mobility, heat over bone
Rx; Preg Cat B (oral) C (IV)

• •

Side Effects
Weight loss
Palpitation
Diarrhea
Tachycardia
Sweating

Nursing Considerations
Used to treat adult hypothyroidism
Side effects are rare and generally associated with overdosing
Dosed at 15mg–30mg initially and titrated up every 2–3 weeks until optimum results are present
Thyroid levels should be checked every 6 months after patient is stabilized
Rx; Preg Cat A

LEVOTHYROXINE (T4)
(lee-voe-thye-<u>rox</u>-een)
(Synthroid, Levothroid)

· ·

Mental Health Medications
ANTI-ANXIETY AGENTS

ALPRAZOLAM
(al-<u>pray</u>-zoe-lam)
(Xanax)

Side Effects
Weight loss
Insomnia, irritability
Nervousness
Arrhythmias, tachycardia

Nursing Considerations
Management of hypothyroidism, myxedema coma, thyroid hormone replacement
PO: peak 1–3 weeks, duration 1–3 weeks
IV: onset 6–8 hours, peak 24 hours
PO: take at same time daily to maintain blood level; take on empty stomach
Do not switch brands unless directed

Avoid OTC meds with iodine and iodized salt, soybeans, tofu, turnips, some seafood, some bread
Drug is not a cure but controls symptoms and treatment is lifelong
Rx; Preg Cat A

• •

Side Effects
Dizziness, drowsiness
Orthostatic hypotension
Blurred vision

Nursing Considerations
Management of anxiety, panic disorders, premenstrual dysphoric disorders
Onset 30 minutes, peak 1–2 hours, duration 4–6 hours
Full therapeutic response takes 2–3 days
May be taken with food
May be habit-forming; do not take for longer than 4 months unless directed
Memory impairment is a sign of long-term use
Do not stop drug abruptly
Drowsiness may worsen at beginning of treatment
Rx; Preg Cat D

BUSPIRONE
(byoo-spye-one)
(BuSpar)

. . . .

CHLORDIAZEPOXIDE
(klor-dye-az-e-pox-ide)
(Librium)

Side Effects

Dizziness, headache,
Stimulation, insomnia,
nervousness
Light-headedness,
numbness
Nausea, diarrhea,
constipation
Tachycardia, palpitations

Nursing Considerations

Management of anxiety
disorders
Onset 7–10 days, optimum
effect may take 3–4 weeks
Use caution with activities
requiring alertness until
response to med is known
Avoid alcohol, other CNS
depressants
Caution when changing
positions, because fainting
may occur, especially in
elderly
Drowsiness may worsen at
beginning of treatment
Rx; Preg Cat B

• •

Side Effects

Dizziness
Drowsiness
Pain at IM site

Nursing Considerations

Management of anxiety
and treatment of alcohol
withdrawal
PO: onset 1–2 hours, peak
1/2–4 hours
IM: onset 15–30 minutes,
slow, erratic absorption
IV: onset 1–5 minutes, duration 15–60 minutes
Use caution with activities
requiring alertness until
response to med is known
Abrupt stop may lead to

withdrawal: insomnia,
irritability, nervousness,
tremors
Avoid alcohol, other CNS
depressants
Tablets may be crushed and
taken with food or fluids for
ease of swallowing
Rx; Schedule C-IV; Preg
Cat D

Mental Health Medications
ANTI-ANXIETY AGENTS

DIAZEPAM
(dye-<u>az</u>-e-pam)

(Valium)

• •

Mental Health Medications
ATTENTION DEFICIT DISORDER AGENTS

METHYLPHENIDATE HCL
(meth-ill-<u>fen</u>-uh-date)

(Concerta)

Side Effects
Drowsiness, fatigue, ataxia
Hypotension
Paradoxic anxiety, especially
in elderly
Orthostatic hypotension
Blurred vision

Nursing Considerations
Treatment of anxiety,
acute alcohol withdrawal,
seizures; pre-operative and
skeletal muscle relaxant
PO: May be taken with
food, onset 1/2 hour
IM: inject deep, slowly into
large muscle mass; inset
15–30 minutes, duration
1–1 1/2 hours, slow and erratic absorption
IV: into large vein, push doses
should not exceed 5 mg/min-
ute, resuscitation equipment
available; onset immediate,
duration 15 minutes–1 hour
Smoking may decrease ef-
fectiveness
Avoid use with alcohol,
other CNS depressants
Long-term use withdrawal
symptoms: vomiting, sweating, abdominal muscle
cramps, tremors, and pos-
sibly convulsions
May be habit-forming if
used over 4 months
Rx; Schedule C-IV; Preg
Cat D

• • • • • • • • • • • • • • • • • • • •

Side Effects
Headache
Respiratory infections
Abdominal pain
Cough

Nursing Considerations
Used to treat attention
deficit disorder (ADHD) in
children over 6 years old
Concerta is time-released
and should be swallowed
whole, not chewed
This prescription can not be
refilled
Dosage is adjusted in 18mg
increments to a maximum
of 54mg/day
Contraindicated in patients
with anxiety, tension, and
glaucoma
This medication may be
habit-forming
Rx; Schedule C-II; Preg
Cat C

LORAZEPAM
(lor-<u>a</u>-ze-pam)
(Ativan)

• •

Mental Health Medications
ANTIDEPRESSANTS, TRICYCLIC

AMITRIPTYLINE
(a-mee-<u>trip</u>-ti-leen)
(Elavil)

Side Effects
Dizziness, drowsiness
Orthostatic hypotension
Blurred vision

Nursing Considerations
Management of anxiety,
irritability in psychiatric or
organic disorders, preopera-
tively, insomnia, adjunct in
endoscopic procedures
PO: onset 30 minutes, peak
1–6 hours
IM: Onset 15–30 minutes,
peak 1–1 1/2 hours
IV: Onset 5–15 minutes,
peak unknown
May be taken with food
May be habit-forming; do
not take for longer than
4 months unless directed
Avoid alcohol, other CNS
depressants
Do not stop drug abruptly
Drowsiness may worsen at
beginning of treatment
Rx; Preg Cat D

• •

Side Effects
Sedation/drowsiness
Blurred vision, dry mouth,
diaphoresis
Postural hypotension, pal-
pitations
Nausea, vomiting, diarrhea
Constipation, urinary reten-
tion
Increased appetite
Sexual dysfunction

Nursing Considerations
Treatment of major depres-
sion
Suicide risk high after
10–14 days due to increased
energy
All antidepressants warn
about suicidal ideation for
individuals under age 24
Avoid use with alcohol
Sun block required
Increase fluid intake
Take dose at bedtime due to
sedative effect
Heavy smokers may require
a larger dose
Use safety precautions with
hazardous activity
Avoid sudden positional
changes, partial hypotension
Rx; Preg Cat C

DOXEPIN
(<u>dox</u>-e-pin)
(Adapin, Sinequan)

• •

IMIPRAMINE
(im-<u>ip</u>-ra-meen)
(Tofranil, Tipramine)

Side Effects
Sedation/drowsiness
Blurred vision, dry mouth, diaphoresis
Postural hypotension, palpitations
Nausea, vomiting, diarrhea
Constipation, urinary retention
Anorexia
Sexual dysfunction

Nursing Considerations
Treatment of major depression, anxiety
Avoid use with alcohol
Suicide risk high after 10–14 days due to increased energy
All antidepressants warn about suicidal ideation for individuals under age 24
Increase fluid intake
Take dose at bedtime, due to sedative effect
Heavy smokers may require a larger dose
Use safety precautions with hazardous activity
Avoid sudden positional changes
Rx; Preg Cat C

• •

Side Effects
Sedation/drowsiness
Dry mouth
Postural hypotension, pal-pitations
Diarrhea
Urinary retention
Anorexia

Nursing Considerations
Treatment of depression, enuresis in children
All antidepressants warn about suicidal ideation for individuals under age 24
Full therapeutic effect may take 2–3 weeks
Drug is dispensed in small amounts at beginning of treatment due to suicide potential
Use safety precautions with hazardous activity
Avoid sudden positional changes
Do not stop abruptly: could cause nausea, malaise, headache
Avoid alcohol, other CNS depressants
Rx; Preg Cat C

NORTRIPTYLINE
(nor-<u>trip</u>-ti-leen)
(Pamelor)

· ·

Mental Health Medications
ANTIDEPRESSANTS, SSRI'S

CITALOPRAM
(sit-<u>al</u>-oh-pram)
(Celexa)

Side Effects

Sedation/drowsiness
Blurred vision, dry mouth, diaphoresis
Postural hypotension, palpitations
Nausea, vomiting, diarrhea
Constipation, urinary retention
Increased appetite
Sexual dysfunction

Nursing Considerations

Treatment of major depression
Avoid use with alcohol, other CNS depressants
Suicide risk high after 10–14 days, due to increased energy
All antidepressants warn about suicidal ideation for individuals under age 24
Increase fluid intake
Take dose at bedtime due to sedative effect
Heavy smokers may require a larger dose
Use safety precautions with hazardous activity
Avoid sudden positional changes, partial hypotension
Women: avoid use if pregnant, breast-feeding
Rx; Preg Cat C

- -

Side Effects

Palpitations, bradycardia
Nausea, vomiting, diarrhea
Decreased appetite
Nervousness, insomnia
Drowsiness

Nursing Considerations

Treatment of major depression
All antidepressants warn about suicidal ideation for individuals under age 24
Take in A.M. to avoid insomnia
Can potentiate effects of digoxin, Coumadin, and Valium
Avoid use with alcohol, other CNS depressants for up to one week after end of therapy
Use caution in potentially hazardous activities
Avoid changing positions (lying, sitting, standing) rapidly
Take consistently at same time of day; therapeutic effects in up to four weeks
Rx; Preg Cat C

ESCITALOPRAM
(ess-sye-<u>tal</u>-oh-pram)
(Lexapro)

• •

FLUOXETINE HCL
(floo-<u>ox</u>-uh-teen)
(Prozac)

Side Effects

Changes in sex drive or
ability
Nausea, diarrhea,
constipation
Increased appetite
Drowsiness

Nursing Considerations

Treatment of depression and
generalized anxiety disorder
All antidepressants warn
about suicidal ideation for
individuals under age 24
May start on lower dosage
and increase after 1 week
Full effects may take up to
4 weeks
Contact prescriber if patient
experiences unusual excite-
ment or hallucinations
Rx; Preg Cat C

• •

Side Effects

Palpitations
Nausea, diarrhea, or
constipation
Decreased appetite with
significant weight loss
Nervousness, insomnia
Urinary retention
Drowsiness
Rash, pruritus, excessive
sweating
Fatigue

Nursing Considerations

Treatment of depression/
OCD, bulimia
All antidepressants warn
about suicidal ideation for
individuals under age 24

Take consistently at same
time of day; full therapeutic
effects may require four
weeks
Can potentiate effects of
digoxin, Coumadin, and
Valium
Used for anorexia, not suicidal or homicidal emotions
Avoid use with alcohol,
other CNS depressants for
up to one week after end of
therapy
Use caution in potentially
hazardous activities
Rx; Preg Cat B

PAROXETINE HCL

(pair-<u>ox</u>-eh-teen)

(Paxil)

• •

SERTRALINE HCL

(<u>sir</u>-trah-leen)

(Zoloft)

Side Effects
Palpitations
Nausea, vomiting, diarrhea, or constipation
Decreased appetite
Nervousness, insomnia

Nursing Considerations
Treatment of anxiety, depression, OCD and social anxiety disorder, panic disorder, PTSD
All antidepressants warn about suicidal ideation for individuals under age 24
Take consistently at same time of day; therapeutic effects in up to four weeks
Avoid use with alcohol, other CNS depressants for up to one week after end of therapy
Use caution in potentially hazardous activities
Rx; Preg Cat D

• •

Side Effects
Headache
Dizziness
Tremor
Insomnia
Nausea, diarrhea
Dry mouth
Male sexual dysfunction

Nursing Considerations
Treatment of depression, OCD, panic disorder with or without agoraphobia, PTSD
All antidepressants warn about suicidal ideation for individuals under age 24
Take consistently at same time of day; therapeutic effects take up to four weeks
Can potentiate effects of digoxin, Coumadin, and Valium
Used for anorexia, not suicidal or homicidal emotions
Avoid use with alcohol, other CNS depressants for up to one week after end of therapy
Use caution in potentially hazardous activities
Rx; Preg Cat B

BUPROPION HCL
(byoo-<u>proe</u>-pee-on)
(Wellbutrin, Zyban, Wellbutrin SR, Wellbutrin XL)

• •

DULOXETINE HCL
(doo-<u>lox</u>-eh-teen)
(Cymbalta)

Side Effects
Agitation
Headache
Dry mouth
Nausea, vomiting
Tremor

Nursing Considerations
Treatment of depression and
smoking cessation
All antidepressants warn
about suicidal ideation for
individuals under age 24
If missed dose for depression, take as soon as possible and space remaining
doses at not less than 4 hour
intervals
If missed dose for smoking
cessation, omit dose
May require gradual reduction before stopping
Avoid use with alcohol,
other CNS depressants for
up to one week after end of
therapy
Use caution in potentially
hazardous activities
Avoid changing positions
(lying, sitting, standing)
rapidly
Rx; Preg Cat B

• •

Side Effects
Nausea, decreased appetite
Dry mouth
Constipation
Fatigue, sleepiness
Increased sweating

Nursing Considerations
Treatment of depression,
anxiety and for manage-
ment of diabetic peripheral
neuropathic pain
All antidepressants warn
about suicidal ideation for
individuals under age 24
Educate patient that most
instances of nausea
improved within 2 weeks
Check blood pressure
periodically
Rx; Preg Cat C

MIRTAZAPINE
(mer-<u>taz</u>-e-peen)
(Remeron)

· ·

TRAZODONE
(<u>tray</u>-zoe-doan)
(Desyrel)

Side Effects
   Drowsiness, dizziness
   Constipation
   Dry mouth
   Increased appetite, weight
   gain

Nursing Considerations
   Treatment of depression
   All antidepressants warn
   about suicidal ideation for
   individuals under age 24
   Do not use within 14 days of
   MAO inhibitor
   May require gradual reduc-
   tion before stopping
   Check with clinician before
   taking OTC cold remedy
   Avoid use with alcohol,
   other CNS depressants for
   up to one week after end of
   therapy
   Use caution in potentially
   hazardous activities
   Rx; Preg Cat C

• •

Side Effects
   Drowsiness
   Hypotension
   Dry mouth
   Nausea
   Dizziness
   Priapism

Nursing Considerations
   Treatment of major
   depression
   All antidepressants warn
   about suicidal ideation for
   individuals under age 24
   Take with or immedi-
   ately after meals to lessen
   GI upset
   If dose missed, take it immediately, unless within

4 hours of next dose
May require gradual reduction before stop
Avoid use with alcohol,
other CNS depressants for
up to one week after end of
therapy
Use caution in potentially
hazardous activities
Avoid changing positions
(lying, sitting, standing)
rapidly
Rx; Preg Cat C

VENLAFAXINE
(ven-lah-<u>fax</u>-een)
(Effexor)

• •

Mental Health Medications
ANTIPSYCHOTICS

HALOPERIDOL
(ha-loe-<u>per</u>-i-dole)
(Haldol)

Side Effects
Abnormal dreams, insomnia
Anxiety, nervousness
Dizziness, weakness
Headache
Abdominal pain
Nausea, vomiting, diarrhea
Anorexia, weight loss
Sexual dysfunction
Sedation

Nursing Considerations
Treatment of major depression or relapse, generalized anxiety disorder
All antidepressants warn about suicidal ideation for individuals under age 24
Take with food; extended release tablets should be swallowed whole
If dose missed, take immediately unless time for next dose
May require gradual reduction before stopping if taken over 6 weeks
Avoid use with alcohol, other CNS depressants for up to one week after end of therapy
Use caution in potentially hazardous activities
Avoid changing positions (lying, sitting, standing) rapidly
Rx; Preg Cat C

• •

Side Effects
Drowsiness
Dizziness

Nursing Considerations
Treatment of psychotic states, Tourette syndrome
PO concentrate: dilute with water, not coffee or tea
PO: Take with food or full glass of water/milk
IM: Inject slowly, deep into UOQ of buttock; have patient lie down for 1/2 hour
Avoid abrupt withdrawal; discontinue gradually
Avoid use with alcohol, other CNS depressants
Use caution in potentially hazardous activities
Avoid changing positions (lying/sitting/standing) rapidly
Wear protective clothing, sunglasses due to photosensitivity
Rx; Preg Cat C

OLANZAPINE
(oh-<u>lan</u>-zuh-peen)
(Zyprexa)

· ·

RISPERIDONE
(riss-<u>pair</u>-i-doan)
(Risperdal)

Side Effects
  Somnolence
  Agitation
  Hostility
  Dizziness
  Rhinitis
  Nervousness
  Joint pain

Nursing Considerations
  Useful in psychotic disorder
  management
  Has been used successfully
  in manic episodes associated with bipolar I
  Use caution when rising
  due to postural hypotension
  possibility
  Dosage should be managed
  tightly when established
  Use caution when operating
  equipment
  Off-label use linked to increased mortality in elderly
  Rx; Preg Cat C

• •

Side Effects
  Drowsiness
  Dizziness
  Tardive dyskinesia
  Constipation

Nursing Considerations
  Treatment of psychotic
  states
  Avoid use with alcohol,
  other CNS depressants
  Use caution in potentially
  hazardous activities
  Avoid changing positions
  (lying/sitting/standing)
  rapidly
  Notify clinician if fever,
  sore throat, bruising/bleed-
  ing, tics/spasms, trembling,
  shuffling gait
  Avoid strenuous exercise in
  hot weather
  Check before taking OTC
  meds
  Rx; Preg Cat C

QUETIAPINE
(kweh-<u>tie</u>-a-peen)
(Seroquel)

• •

ZIPRASIDONE HCL
(zye-<u>praz</u>-i-doan)
(Geodon)

Side Effects
Drowsiness
Dizziness

Nursing Considerations
Used in treatment of psychotic states
Avoid use with alcohol, other CNS depressants
Use caution in potentially hazardous activities
Avoid changing positions (lying/sitting/standing) rapidly
Notify clinician if fever, sore throat, bruising/bleeding, tics/spasms, trembling, shuffling gait
Avoid strenuous exercise in hot weather
Check before taking OTC meds
Rx; Preg Cat C

• •

Side Effects
Drowsiness
Dizziness
Tardive dyskinesia
Constipation

Nursing Considerations
Used in treatment of psychotic states
Avoid use with alcohol, other CNS depressants
Use caution in potentially hazardous activities
Avoid changing positions (lying/sitting/standing) rapidly
Notify clinician if fever, sore throat, bruising/bleeding, tics/spasms, trembling, shuffling gait
Avoid strenuous exercise in hot weather
Check before taking OTC meds
Women: avoid breastfeeding
Rx; Preg Cat C

CARBAMAZEPINE
(kar-ba-<u>maz</u>-e-peen)
(Tegretol, Tegretol XR)

· ·

DIVALPROEX SODIUM
(dye-<u>val</u>-proe-ex)
(Depakote)

Side Effects
Myelosuppression
Dizziness, drowsiness
Ataxia
Diplopia, rash
Photosensitivity

Nursing Considerations
Management of bipolar
disorder, seizures,
trigeminal neuralgia, diabetic neuropathy
Avoid driving and other
activities requiring alertness
the first 3 days
Monitor blood levels, CBC
regularly, esp. during first
2 months; periodic eye
exams

Take with food or milk to
decrease GI upset; tablets
(non extended release) may
be crushed, extended release
capsules may be opened,
mixed with juice or soft
food
Urine may turn pink to
brown
Avoid abrupt withdrawal;
discontinue gradually
Avoid use with alcohol,
other CNS depressants
Patient should wear medical
information tag
Rx; Preg Cat C

• •

Side Effects
Sedation, drowsiness,
dizziness
Mental status and
behavioral changes
Nausea, vomiting, constipa-
tion, diarrhea, heartburn
Prolonged bleeding time

Nursing Considerations
Management of seizures,
manic episodes associated
with bipolar disorder (delayed release only), migraine
prophylaxis (delayed and
extended release only)
Take with or immedi-
ately after meals to lessen
GI upset

Swallow tablets or capsules
whole (no crushing, chewing)
Avoid abrupt withdrawal
after long-term use; discontinue gradually to prevent
convulsions
Monitor blood levels, platelets, bleeding time, and liver
function tests
Delayed release products:
peak blood level 3–5 hours,
duration: 12–24 hours
Extended release products:
peak blood level 7–14 hours,
duration: 24 hours
Wear medical information
tag
Rx; Preg Cat D

LITHIUM
(<u>li</u>-thee-um)
(Lithobid, Eskalith)

. . . .

TEMAZEPAM
(tem-<u>as</u>-eh-pam)
(Restoril)

Side Effects
  Dizziness
  Impaired vision
  Fine hand tremors
  Reversible leukocytosis
  Signs of intoxication: vomiting, diarrhea, drowsiness, muscular weakness, ataxia

Nursing Considerations
  Controls manic episodes in manic depressive individuals; mood stabilizer
  Use caution in potentially hazardous activities
  Check serum levels 2 times weekly during treatment, q 2–3 mos on maintenance; draw blood in A.M. prior to dose

  Target serum levels: treatment = .5–1.5 mEq/L, maintenance = .6–1.2mEq/L
  GI symptoms reduced if taken with meals
  Onset of therapeutic effects in 1–2 weeks
  Diabetics: closely monitor blood/urine glucose
  Dose reduced during depressive stages of illness
  Encourage 10–12 glasses H_2O/day and adequate salt intake (6–10 grams/day)
  Avoid caffeine, increased exercise, saunas
  Rx; Preg Cat D

• •

Side Effects
  Drowsiness
  Dizziness
  Lethargy
  Weakness
  Euphoria
  Anorexia

Nursing Considerations
  Used for short-term (7–10 days) treatment of insomnia
  Should be avoided in patients under the age of 18
  Avoid alcohol while taking this drug
  Not intended for use for more than 10 days
  When used with CNS depressants, the CNS depression is increased
  Rx; Schedule C-IV; Preg Cat D

ZALEPION
(zuh-lay-<u>pee</u>-own)
(Sonata)

• •

ZOLPIDEM TRARTRATE
(<u>zol</u>-puh-dim)
(Ambien)

Side Effects
- Headache
- Myalgia
- Dizziness
- Asthenia
- Dyspepsia
- Eye pain

Nursing Considerations
Used in short-term insomnia treatment

Zalepion does not prolong sleep time or decrease awakenings

Elderly patients generally benefit the most

Because of rapid onset, patients should take immediately before bedtime

Avoid alcohol while using this medication

May be habit-forming

Rx; Schedule C-IV; Preg Cat C

• •

Side Effects
- Headache
- Drowsiness
- Dizziness
- Influenza-like symptoms
- Nausea

Nursing Considerations
Short-term treatment of insomnia

Dosage may need to be adjusted down if patient is using a CNS-depressant to avoid an addictive effect

Side effects increase with prolonged usage

Rx; Preg Cat B

ALLOPURINOL
(al-oh-<u>pure</u>-i-nole)
(Aloprim, Zyloprim)

. . . .

COLCHICINE
(<u>kol</u>-chi-seen)

Side Effects
GI upset
Headache, drowsiness
Rash

Nursing Considerations
Treatment of gout, uric acid
neuropathy, uric acid stone
formation
Encourage 10–12 glasses
H_2O/day
Check CBC and renal
function tests
Take with food; don't take
Vitamin C or iron
Initial therapy can increase
attacks
Avoid use of alcohol, eating
organ meats, gravy, legumes
Full therapeutic effect may
require several months
Rx; Preg Cat C

• •

Side Effects
Nausea, vomiting, diarrhea
Agranulocytosis
Sign of toxicity: abdominal
cramps

Nursing Considerations
Treatment and prevention
of acute gout attacks
Has analgesic, anti-inflam-
matory effects
Take with food/milk
IV: slowly; do not administer
IM/subQ
Encourage 10–12 glasses
H_2O/day
Avoid use of alcohol, eating
organ meats, gravy, legumes
Always carry medication to
treat acute attacks
Rx; Preg Cat D

PROBENECID
(proe-<u>ben</u>-e-sid)
(Benemid)

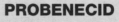

Musculoskeletal Medications
NONSALICYLATE NSAIDS, ANTIRHEUMATICS

DICLOFENAC NA
(dye-<u>kloe</u>-fen-ak)
(Voltaren)

Side Effects	Nursing Considerations
Nausea	Treatment of hyperurice-mia assoc. with gout, gouty arthritis
Skin rash	
Hemolytic anemia	
Sore gums, anorexia	Check BUN, renal function tests
	Encourage 8–10 glasses H_2O/day
	Give with milk, food, and antacids
	Avoid use of alcohol, eating organ meats, gravy, legumes
	Avoid aspirin-containing products, may take acet-aminophen
	Rx; Preg Cat B

• •

Side Effects	Nursing Considerations
Dizziness	Used in arthritic conditions, dysmenorrhea
Headache	
Nephrotoxicity	Ophthalmic: reduce in-flammation after cataract extraction
Blood dyscrasias	
	PO: Take with full glass of water and food and remain upright for 1/2 hour
	If dose missed, take within 2 hours
	Use sunscreen to prevent photosensitivity
	Awareness of increased risk of heart attack or stroke (all nonsalicylate NSAIDS)
	Rx; Preg Cat B

ETODOLAC
(ee-<u>toe</u>-doe-lak)

(Lodine)

· ·

IBUPROFEN
(eye-byoo-<u>proe</u>-fen)

(Advil, Motrin)

Side Effects
- Nephrotoxicity
- Nausea
- Anorexia
- Dizziness
- Blood dyscrasias

Nursing Considerations
Reduces pain of osteoarthritis
Monitor for signs of toxicity: blurred vision, ringing or roaring in ears
Full therapeutic effect may take up to 1 month
Avoid concurrent use of ASA, NSAIDs, acetaminophen, alcohol
Awareness of increased risk of heart attack or stroke (all nonsalicylate NSAIDS)
Rx; Preg Cat C

- -

Side Effects
- Nausea, vomiting, diarrhea, constipation
- Headache, dizziness
- Fluid retention

Nursing Considerations
Treatment of rheumatoid arthritis/osteoarthritis; relief of mild/moderate pain; antipyretic
Take with milk or food
Use cautiously with aspirin allergy
Awareness of increased risk of heart attack or stroke (all nonsalicylate NSAIDS)
Rx/OTC; Preg Cat C, contraindicated in third trimester

INDOMETHACIN
(in-doe-<u>meth</u>-a-sin)
(Indocin)

• •

MELOXICAM
(mell-<u>ox</u>-i-kam)
(Mobic)

Side Effects	Nursing Considerations
Peptic ulcer	Treatment of rheumatoid arthritis/osteoarthritis, acute gout, acute painful shoulder
Dizziness	
Bone marrow depression	
Drowsiness	
Blurred vision	Observe for bleeding problems
	PO: Take with food/milk, encourage upright position for 15–30 minutes
	Use caution with potentially hazardous activities
	Avoid use with alcohol, aspirin, other NSAIDs
	Awareness of increased risk of heart attack or stroke (all nonsalicylate NSAIDs)
	Rx; Preg Cat C

• •

Side Effects	Nursing Considerations
Diarrhea, constipation, gas	Relief of pain, tenderness and stiffness of osteoarthritis, rheumatoid arthritis and juvenile rheumatoid arthritis
Sore throat, cough, runny nose	
	Awareness of increased risk of heart attack or stroke (all nonsalicylate NSAIDS)
	Rx; Preg Cat C

PIROXICAM
(peer-<u>ox</u>-i-kam)

(Feldene)

• •

Musculoskeletal Medications
SALICYLATES, ANTIRHEUMATICS

SALSALATE
(<u>sal</u>-sah-late)

(Disalcid)

Side Effects
  Drowsiness
  Headache

Nursing Considerations
  For mild to moderate pain
  PO: with food to decrease
  GI upset; on empty stomach
  to increase absorption
  Take at same time every day
  Monitor for signs of toxic-
  ity: blurred vision, ringing
  or roaring in ears
  Full therapeutic effect may
  take up to 1 month
  Avoid concurrent use of
  ASA, other OTC meds,
  alcohol
  Awareness of increased risk
  of heart attack or stroke (all
  nonsalicylate NSAIDs)
  Rx; Preg Cat B

• •

Side Effects
  Nausea, vomiting
  GI bleeding
  Heartburn
  Rash

Nursing Considerations
  For mild to moderate pain
  PO: can be crushed or
  whole
  PO: take with food or milk
  to decrease GI upset
  Full therapeutic effect may
  take 2 weeks
  Read label on OTC meds,
  may contain ASA
  Monitor for signs of toxic-
  ity: changes in liver, kidney,
  eye, ear functions
  Rx; Preg Cat C

BACLOFEN
(<u>bak</u>-loe-fen)
(Lioresal)

• •

CARISOPRODOL
(kar-eye-soe-<u>proe</u>-dole)
(Soma)

Side Effects
- Drowsiness
- Dizziness
- Weakness, fatigue
- Confusion
- Nausea, vomiting

Nursing Considerations
- Used to reduce spasticity in multiple sclerosis, spinal cord injury
- Take with food
- Avoid alcohol, other CNS depressants
- Increased risk of seizures in patients with seizure disorder
- Withdraw gradually over 1–2 weeks, unless severe adverse reactions; D/C may cause hallucinations, tachycardia or rebound spasticity
- Monitor for symptoms of sensitivity: fever, skin eruptions, respiratory distress
- Rx; Preg Cat C

• •

Side Effects
- Drowsiness
- Dizziness
- Light-headedness
- Nausea

Nursing Considerations
- Relief of pain, stiffness
- PO: onset 1/2 hour, peak 4 hours, duration 4–6 hours
- Avoid alcohol, other CNS depressants, including OTC cold or allergy meds
- Avoid activities requiring alertness until effects known
- Rx; Preg Cat C

CYCLOBENZAPRINE
(sye-kole-<u>ben</u>-za-preen)
(Flexeril)

· ·

METAXALONE
(meh-<u>tax</u>-uh-lone)
(Skelaxin)

Side Effects
  Drowsiness
  Dizziness
  Dry mouth
  Constipation

Nursing Considerations
  Relieves muscle spasms
  from acute conditions
  Avoid alcohol, other CNS
  depressants, including OTC
  cold or allergy meds
  Avoid activities requiring
  alertness until effects known
  Rx; Preg Cat B

• •

Side Effects
  Drowsiness
  Dizziness
  Headache
  Gastrointestinal pains

Nursing Considerations
  Used to relieve painful
  musculoskeletal injuries
  Should be an adjunct to rest
  and physical therapy
  Avoid alcohol while using
  this drug
  Use caution when operating
  machinery
  Use cautiously in patients
  with known liver
  impairment
  Rx; Preg Cat C

METHOCARBAMOL
(meth-oh-<u>kar</u>-ba-mole)
(Robaxin)

• •

Neurological Medications
Neurological Medications

BENZTROPINE
(<u>benz</u>-troe-peen)
(Cogentin)

Side Effects
Drowsiness
Dizziness
Light-headedness
Nausea

Nursing Considerations
Relieves muscle spasms
from acute conditions,
tetanus management
IM: Inject deep into UOQ of
buttock, rotate sites
NG tube: Crush tablets into
fluid
PO: Take with food or milk
Metallic taste may develop
Urine may turn green, black
or brown
Avoid alcohol, other CNS
depressants, including OTC
cold or allergy meds
Avoid activities requiring
alertness until effects known
Rx; Preg Cat C

• •

Side Effects
Dry mouth
Constipation

Nursing Considerations
Treatment of Parkinson
symptoms, EPS associated
with neuroleptic drugs,
acute dystonic reactions
IM/IV: onset 15 minutes,
duration 6–10 hours
PO: onset 1 hour, duration
6–10 hours
Tablets may be crushed and
mixed with food
Taper med over a week, or
withdrawal symptoms: EPS,
tremors, insomnia, tachy-
cardia, restlessness

Avoid hazardous activities
until stabilized on med
Change positions slowly
Avoid alcohol, antihista-
mines unless directed
Rx; Preg Cat C

CAFFEINE/ERGOTAMINE
(er-<u>got</u>-a-meen)
(Cafergot)

• •

CARBIDOPA/LEVODOPA
(<u>leev</u>-oe-doe-pa)
(Sinemet)

Side Effects
- Headache
- Tremors, convulsions
- Blood vessel contraction, with decreased circulation, especially limbs
- Toxic ergotism: nausea, vomiting, diarrhea, dizziness, headache, mental confusion

Nursing Considerations
- Treatment of vascular headache
- Take at onset of pain/during prodomal stage to abort headache
- Lie down in darkened quiet room for several hours
- Rx; Preg Cat X

Side Effects
- Twitching
- Headache, dizziness
- Dark urine/sweat
- Cardiac arrhythmias
- Mental changes: confusion, agitation, mood alterations

Nursing Considerations
- Replacement dopaminergic agent
- Change positions slowly
- Take with food, decreased effect with liver, pork, wheat germ, and vitamin B6
- Full therapeutic effect may take several months
- Rx; Preg Cat C

DONEPEZIL
(don-ep-<u>ee</u>-zill)

(Aricept)

• •

LEVODOPA
(<u>leev</u>-oe-doe-pa)

(Dopar, Larodopa)

Side Effects
- Nausea, vomiting, diarrhea
- Headache
- Insomnia
- Seizures

Nursing Considerations
Used in treatment of mild to
moderate dementia
Drug does not cure but sta-
bilizes or relieves symptoms
Take at regular intervals
Take between meals or
may be given with meals to
decrease GI upset
Rx; Preg Cat C

• •

Side Effects
- Twitching
- Headache, dizziness
- Dark urine/sweat
- Cardiac arrhythmias
- Mental changes: confusion,
  agitation, mood alterations

Nursing Considerations
Replacement dopaminergic
agent
Change positions slowly
Take with food, decreased
effect with liver, pork, wheat
germ and vitamin B6
Full therapeutic effect may
take several weeks to a few
months
Rx; Preg Cat C

METHYLPHENIDATE
(meth-ill-<u>fen</u>-i-date)
(Ritalin)

• •

SELEGILINE
(se-<u>le</u>-ji-leen)
(Eldepryl)

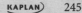

Side Effects
Hyperactivity, insomnia
Restlessness, talkativeness
Palpitations, tachycardia

Nursing Considerations
Management of attention
deficit hyperactive disorder,
narcolepsy, depression in
the elderly
Onset 1/2 hour, duration
4–6 hours
Take at least 6 hours before
bedtime (regular release)
or 10 hours before bedtime
(sustained release, extended
release)
Taper med over several
weeks, or depression, in-
creased sleeping, lethargy
will occur
Avoid hazardous activities
until stabilized on med
Decrease caffeine consumption (coffee, tea, cola, choco-
late) to decrease irritability
Rx; Schedule C-II; Preg
Cat C

• •

Side Effects
Dizziness
Cardiac dysrhythmias

Nursing Considerations
Indirect acting dopaminergic agent
Used in management of
Parkinson's disease with
levodopa/carbidopa
Do not use with tricyclics or
opioids
Monitor for signs of toxicity: twitching, eye spasms
Do not stop abruptly; par-
kinsonian crisis may occur
Avoid foods high in tyra-
mine: cheese, pickled products, alcohol, large amounts
of caffeine
Rx; Preg Cat C

ZOLMITRIPTAN
(zole-mih-<u>trip</u>-tan)
(Zomig)

. . . .

Opthalmics
ANTIGLAUCOMA MEDICATIONS

DORZOLAMIDE HCL
(dor-<u>zoh</u>-la-mide)
(Trusopt)

Side Effects

Weakness, neck stiffness
Tingling, hot sensation,
burning, feeling of pressure,
tightness
Numbness, dizziness,
sedation

Nursing Considerations

Used for treatment of acute
migraine with or without
aura
Take with fluids as soon as
symptoms occur
PO: Tablet may be split
Avoid foods high in tyra-
mine: cheese, pickled products, alcohol, large amounts
of caffeine
Rx; Preg Cat C

• •

Side Effects

Ocular burning, stinging,
discomfort
Blurred vision, tearing, or
dryness
Photophobia
Bitter taste in mouth

Nursing Considerations

Treatment of glaucoma and
ocular hypertension
Wash hands before and after
instillation
Do not touch tip of dropper
to eye or body
Do not wear contact lens
during instillation
Drug is a sulfonamide.
Although given topically, it
can be absorbed
systemically
Stop if eye inflammation or
eyelid reactions
Rx; Preg Cat C

DORZOLAMIDE/TIMOLOL
(dor-<u>zoh</u>-la-mide <u>tye</u>-moe-lole)
(Cosopt)

• •

TRAVOPROST
(<u>trav</u>-oh-prahst)
(Travatan)

Side Effects

Ocular burning, stinging, discomfort

Blurred vision, tearing, or dryness

Photophobia

Bitter taste in mouth

Nursing Considerations

Treatment of glaucoma and ocular hypertension

Place pressure on tear ducts for one minute

Wash hands before and after instillation

Do not touch drug container to eye or body

Do not wear contact lens during instillation

Drug contains sulfonamide. Although given topically, it can be absorbed systemically

Stop if eye inflammation or eyelid reactions

Rx; Preg Cat C

• •

Side Effects

Ocular hyperemia

Decreased visual acuity

Eye discomfort or pain

Foreign body sensation

Eye pruritus

Nursing Considerations

Treatment of glaucoma and ocular hypertension for patient who can't tolerate or responds inadequately to other IOP-lowering drugs

Place pressure on tear ducts for one minute

Wash hands before and after instillation

Do not touch tip of dropper to eye or body

Potential for increased brown pigmentation of iris, eyelid skin darkening, changes in eyelashes, important if only one eye being treated

Stop if eye inflammation or eyelid reactions

Remove contact lens to give med, can reinsert in 15 minutes

Discard med six months after opening

Rx; Preg Cat C

LEVOBUNOLOL
(lee-voe-<u>byoo</u>-no-lole)
(Ak-beta, Betagan)

• •

TIMOLOL
(<u>tim</u>-oh-lole)
(Timoptic gel, Betimol solution)

Side Effects
  Hypotension
  Transient eye stinging and
  burning
  Asthma attacks in patients
  with history of asthma

Nursing Considerations
  Treatment of glaucoma and
  ocular hypertension
  Place pressure on tear ducts
  for one minute
  Wash hands before and after
  instillation
  Do not touch tip of dropper
  to eye or body
  Drug is a beta blocker.
  Although given topically, it
  can be absorbed
  systemically
  Report shortness of breath,
  chest pain or heart
  irregularity
  Wear medical identification tag
  Rx; Preg Cat C

• •

Side Effects
  Fatigue
  Weakness

Nursing Considerations
  Treatment of glaucoma and
  ocular hypertension
  Place pressure on tear ducts
  for one minute
  Wash hands before and after
  instillation
  Do not touch drug con-
  tainer to eye or body
  Rx; Preg Cat C

BRIMONIDINE TARTRATE
(brih-<u>moh</u>-nih-deen)
(Alphagan)

• •

CROMOLYN NA
(<u>kroe</u>-moe-lin)
(Opticrom)

Side Effects
  Ocular hyperemia
  Allergic conjunctivitis
  Pruritus

Nursing Considerations
  Treatment of glaucoma and
  ocular hypertension
  Wait 15 minutes after use to
  wear soft contact lens
  Use caution with hazardous
  activities due to decreased
  mental alertness
  Avoid alcohol
  Monitor intraocular pressure because may reverse
  after 1 month of therapy
  Rx; Preg Cat B

• •

Side Effects
  Ocular irritation

Nursing Considerations
  Used in treatment of con-
  junctivitis, keratitis
  Wash hands before and after
  instillation
  Do not touch tip of dropper
  to eye or body
  Do not wear soft contact
  lens while using this med
  Rx; Preg Cat B

FLURBIPROFEN
(flur-bi-<u>proe</u>-fen)
(Ocufen)

• •

ANTIPYRINE/BENZOCAINE/GLYCERIN OTIC SOLUTION
(Auralgan)

Side Effects
Ocular irritation

Nursing Considerations
Inhibition of intraoperative miosis
Give every half hour, starting 2 hours before surgery, 4 drops to each eye
Rx; Preg Cat C

• •

Nursing Considerations
Otic analgesic
Suspension: shake well (also comes in solution)
Can warm up with hands for patient's comfort
Warn patient not to touch ear with dropper
Warn patient that drug is for use only in ears
Rx; Preg Cat C

HYDROCORTISONE/NEOMYCIN/
POLYMIXIN OTIC
(Cortisporin)

● ●

Respiratory Medications
ANTIASTHMAS, OTHER

ALBUTEROL/IPRATROPIUM INHALER
(al-<u>byoo</u>-tear-ol/eye-pra-<u>troe</u>-pee-um)
(Combivent)

Nursing Considerations
Otic analgesic and antibiotic
Warn patient not to touch
ear with dropper
Explain drug is for use only
in ears
Rx; Preg Cat C

- -

Side Effects
Nervousness, hyperactivity
Tremors
Dry mouth, photophobia,
constipation
Tachycardia, palpitations
Nausea, vomiting
Headache

Nursing Considerations
Treatment of asthma
Teach how to correctly use
inhaler
Monitor for toxicity
Assess for hypersensitiv-
ity, including soy products,
atropine, peanuts
Encourage 10–12 glasses
H_2O/day
Avoid OTC cough/hayfever
medications
Use caution with hazardous
activities
Rx; Preg Cat C

CROMOLYN SODIUM INHALER
(<u>kroe</u>-moe-lin)
(Intal)

· ·

MONTELUKAST
(mon-tea-<u>lew</u>-cast)
(Singulair)

Side Effects
  Bronchospasm
  Cough
  Dizziness

Nursing Considerations
  Treatment of asthma
  Notify clinician of wheez-
  ing, respiratory distress
  Do not use for acute asthma
  attacks
  Full therapeutic effect may
  take several weeks
  Rx; Preg Cat B

• •

Side Effects
  Dizziness
  Headache

Nursing Considerations
  Prophylaxis and treatment
  of chronic asthma
  Do not use to treat acute
  symptoms; use a rapid-acting bronchodilator
  Notify clinician of wheezing, respiratory distress
  Full therapeutic effect may
  take several weeks
  Rx; Preg Cat B

THEOPHYLLINE
(thee-<u>off</u>-i-lin)
(Theo-Dur, Theovent)

. . . .

BENZONATATE
(ben-<u>zoe</u>-na-tate)
(Tessalon)

Side Effects
Restlessness
Dizziness
Palpitations, sinus tachy-
cardia
Anorexia

Nursing Considerations
Treatment of bronchial
asthma, bronchospasm of
COPD, chronic bronchitis,
emphysema
PO: peak 2 hours; take with
full glass of water; best on
empty stomach
Solution: peak 1 hour
Check all OTC and other
meds for ephedrine before
taking with this med

Avoid alcohol, caffeine,
smoking
Avoid activities requiring
alertness until response to
med is known
Contact clinician if toxicity:
nausea, vomiting, anxiety,
insomnia, convulsions
Drink 8–10 glasses of fluid
per day
Do not crush enteric-coated
SR preparations, swallow
whole
Rx; Preg Cat C

- -

Side Effects
Dizziness
Drowsiness

Nursing Considerations
Treatment of nonproductive
cough
PO: onset 15–20 minutes,
duration 3–8 hours
Capsules should be swal-
lowed whole; do not chew,
because release of med may
cause local anesthetic effect
and choking
Additive CNS depression
may occur with antihista-
mines, alcohol, opioids, and
sedative/hypnotics
Avoid activities requiring

alertness until response to
med is known
Contact clinician if signs
of overdose: convulsions,
trembling, restlessness
Rx; Preg Cat C

HYDROCODONE
(hye-droe-<u>koe</u>-done)
(Hycodan, with acetaminophen Vicodin)

• •

IPRATROPIUM BROMIDE
(eye-pra-<u>troe</u>-pee-um)
(Atrovent)

Side Effects
Nausea, vomiting
Anorexia
Constipation
Circulatory and respiratory
depression
Drowsiness

Nursing Considerations
Treatment of hyperactive
and nonproductive cough,
mild pain relief
Physical dependency may
result when used for ex-
tended periods
Withdrawal symptoms may
occur: nausea, vomiting,
cramps, fever, faintness,
anorexia
Avoid other CNS depres-
sants
Onset: 10–20 minutes, duration 4–6 hours
Rx; Preg Cat C

• •

Side Effects
Nervousness
Tremors
Dry mouth
Palpitations

Nursing Considerations
Treatment of bronchospasm
assoc. with COPD, rhinor-
rhea, rhinitis
Not for acute bronchospasm
needing rapid response
Teach use of metered dose
inhaler: inhale, hold breath,
exhale slowly
Don't mix in nebulizer with
cromolyn sodium
Assess for hypersensitiv-
ity, including soy products,

atropine, peanuts
Encourage 10–12 glasses
H_2O/day
Avoid OTC cough/hayfever
medications
Use caution with hazardous
activities
Rx; Preg Cat B

ALBUTEROL SULFATE
(al-<u>byoo</u>-tear-ol)
(Proventil, Ventolin)

• •

SALMETEROL
(sal-<u>me</u>-te-role)
(Serevent)

Side Effects
Tremors
Headache
Hyperactivity
Tachycardia
Nausea, vomiting

Nursing Considerations
Treatment of bronchial
asthma, reversible bronchospasm
Teach how to correctly use
inhaler
Monitor for toxicity
PO: Take with food to de-
crease GI upset; may crush
tablets
Teach how to take radial
pulse
Rx; Preg Cat C

• •

Side Effects
Headache

Nursing Considerations
Long-term control of asthma, prevention of exercise-
induced asthma, prevention
of bronchospasm in COPD
Do not use to treat acute
symptoms; use a rapid-acting bronchodilator
Contact clinician if dif-
ficulty breathing, if more
inhalations are needed of
rapid-acting bronchodila-
tor or using more than 4
inhalations of a rapid-acting
bronchodilator for 2 or more
consecutive days or more
than 1 canister in 8 weeks
Rx; Preg Cat C

TERBUTALINE SULFATE
(ter-<u>byoo</u>-ta-leen)
(Brethine, Bricanyl)

• •

GUAIFENESIN
(gwye-<u>fen</u>-e-sin)
(Robitussin, Mytussin)

Side Effects
Nervousness
Restlessness
Tremor

Nursing Considerations
Management of asthma or COPD
Inhalation and subQ used for short-term control; PO as long-term
PO: take with food to decrease GI upset
Tablets may be crushed and mixed with food or fluids
SubQ: Give injections in lateral deltoid
Contact clinician if unrelieved shortness of breath
Rx; Preg Cat B

• •

Side Effects
Nausea

Nursing Considerations
Treatment of dry, nonproductive cough
PO: onset 30 minutes, duration 4–6 hours
PO extended release: duration 12 hours
OTC/Rx; Preg Cat C

CROMOLYN SODIUM
(<u>kroe</u>-moe-lin)
(Nasalcrom)

· ·

Treatment/Replacement
ALCOHOL DETERRENTS

DISULFIRAM
(dye-<u>sul</u>-fih-ram)
(Antabuse)

Side Effects
  Nasal burning and irritation
  Headache
  Bad taste
  Epistaxis
  Postnasal drip

Nursing Considerations
  Prophylaxis and treatment
  of allergic rhinitis
  Full therapeutic effect may
  take several weeks
  Rx; Preg Cat B

• •

Side Effects
  In the absence of alcohol:
  drowsiness, headache, restlessness, fatigue
  In the presence of alcohol:
  flushing, chest pain, heart
  arrythmias, hypotension,
  seizures, throbbing in head
  and neck, sweating

Nursing Considerations
  Used for treatment of
  chronic alcoholism by caus-
  ing severe hypersensitivity
  Onset may be delayed up to
  12 hours; single dose may be
  effective for 1–2 weeks
  Never give without patient's
  knowledge
  Avoid alcohol in any form:
  in foods, sauces, or other
  meds, such as cough syrups
  or tonics
  Avoid vinegar, paregoric,
  skin products, liniments or
  lotions containing alcohol
  Wear medical information
  tag
  Rx; Preg Cat C

CARBONYL IRON
(Feosol)

• •

FERRIC GLUCONATE COMPLEX
(Ferriecit)

Side Effects
  Nausea, constipation
  Epigastric pain
  Black and red tarry stools

Nursing Considerations
  Treatment of iron deficiency anemia, prophylaxis for iron deficiency in pregnancy
  Contains 100% elemental iron
  Keep upright for 15–30 minutes to avoid esophageal corrosion, take 1 hour before bedtime
  Stools will become black or dark green
  Take on empty stomach, not with antacids or milk
  Do not substitute one iron salt for another, since iron content differs
  Rx; Preg Cat B

• •

Side Effects
  Nausea, constipation
  Epigastric pain
  Black and red tarry stools

Nursing Considerations
  Treatment of iron deficiency anemia in dialysis patients, given IV
  Onset 4 days, peak 1–2 weeks
  Stools will become black or dark green
  Rx; Preg Cat C

FERROUS FUMARATE
(Femiron, Feostat)

• •

FERROUS GLUCONATE
(Fergon)

Side Effects
Nausea, constipation
Epigastric pain
Black and red tarry stools

Nursing Considerations
Treatment of iron deficiency anemia, prophylaxis for iron deficiency in pregnancy
Contains 33% elemental iron
Keep upright for 15–30 minutes to avoid esophageal corrosion, take 1 hour before bedtime
Stools will become black or dark green
Take on empty stomach, not with antacids or milk
Do not substitute one iron salt for another, since iron content differs
Rx; Preg Cat B

• •

Side Effects
Nausea, constipation
Epigastric pain
Black and red tarry stools

Nursing Considerations
Treatment of iron deficiency anemia, prophylaxis for iron deficiency in pregnancy
Contains 12% elemental iron
Keep upright for 15–30 minutes to avoid esophageal corrosion, take 1 hour before bedtime
Stools will become black or dark green
Take on empty stomach, not with antacids or milk
Do not substitute one iron salt for another, since iron content differs
Rx; Preg Cat B

FERROUS SULFATE
(Feosol)

• •

IRON POLYSACCHARIDE
(Niferex)

Side Effects
Nausea, constipation
Epigastric pain
Black and red tarry stools

Nursing Considerations
Treatment of iron deficiency anemia, prophylaxis for iron deficiency in pregnancy
Contains 30% elemental iron
Keep upright for 15–30 minutes to avoid esophageal corrosion, take 1 hour before bedtime
Stools will become black or dark green
Take on empty stomach, not with antacids or milk
Do not substitute one iron salt for another, since iron content differs
Rx; Preg Cat B

• •

Side Effects
Nausea, constipation
Epigastric pain
Black and red tarry stools

Nursing Considerations
Treatment of iron deficiency anemia, prophylaxis for iron deficiency in pregnancy
Keep upright for 15–30 minutes to avoid esophageal corrosion, take 1 hour before bedtime
Stools will become black or dark green
Take on empty stomach, not with antacids or milk
Do not substitute one iron salt for another, since iron content differs
Rx; Preg Cat B

POTASSIUM
(K-Lor)

NALOXONE HCL
(nal-<u>ox</u>-own)
(Narcan)

Side Effects
  Nausea, vomiting
  Cramps, diarrhea

Nursing Considerations
  Prevention and treatment of
  hypocalemia
  Onset for PO 30 minutes,
  IV immediate
  Do not give IM, subQ
  Avoid OTC antacids, salt
  substitutes, analgesics, vita-
  mins unless directed
  Report hyperkalemia: lethargy, confusion, GI symptoms, fainting, decreased
  output
  Report continued hypo-
  calemia: fatigue, weakness,
  polyuria, polydipsia, cardiac
  changes
  OTC/Rx; Preg Cat C

• •

Side Effects
  Withdrawal symptoms
  in narcotic-dependent
  patients: restlessness, muscle
  spasms, tearing

Nursing Considerations
  Used to reverse narcotic
  depression, including respiratory symptoms
  IM and subQ onset in 2 to 5
  minutes; IV 1 to 2 minutes
  Have emergency support
  equipment available
  Rx; Preg Cat B

CHOLECALCIFEROL (VITAMIN D$_3$)
ERGOCALCIFEROL (VITAMIN D$_2$)
(kole-e-kal-<u>sif</u>-e-role, er-goe-kal-<u>sif</u>-e-role)
(Calderol, Caldiferol)

• •

CYANOCOBALAMIN
(sye-an-oh-koe-<u>bal</u>-a-min)
(Cobex, Crystamine, Cyomin)

Side Effects
Metallic taste, dry mouth

Nursing Considerations
Treatment of Vitamin D
deficiency, rickets, psoriasis,
rheumatoid arthritis
If med missed, omit
Decrease use of antacids
and laxatives containing
magnesium
Rx; Preg Cat C

• •

Side Effects
Diarrhea

Nursing Considerations
Treatment of Vitamin B_{12}
deficiency, pernicious anemia, hemorrhage, renal and
hepatic disease
IM, subQ, nasal: peak 3–10
days
Foods high in this vitamin:
meats, seafood, egg yolk,
fermented cheeses
Excessive intake of alcohol
or vitamin C may decrease
oral absorption/effectiveness
OTC/Rx; Preg Cat A

FOLIC ACID
(<u>foe</u>-lik <u>a</u>-cid)

• •

HYDROXOCOBALAMIN
(hye-<u>drox</u>-o-ko-bal-a-min)

(Vibral, Vitamin B$_{12}$)

Side Effects
Bronchospasm

Nursing Considerations
Treatment of anemia, liver disease, alcoholism, intestinal obstruction, pregnancy
Also contained in bran, yeast, dried beans, nuts, fruits, fresh vegetables, asparagus
OTC; Preg Cat A

• •

Side Effects
Diarrhea

Nursing Considerations
Treatment of Vitamin B_{12} deficiency, pernicious anemia, hemorrhage, renal and hepatic disease
IM, subQ: peak 3–10 days
Foods high in this vitamin: meats, seafood, egg yolk, fermented cheeses
OTC/Rx; Preg Cat A

NIACINAMIDE
(nye-ah-<u>sin</u>-ah-myd)

• •

Women's Health
CONTRACEPTIVES, SYSTEMIC

DESOGESTREL/ETHINYL ESTRADIOL
(dess-oh-<u>jes</u>-trel <u>eth</u>-in-il es-tra-<u>dye</u>-ole)
(Cyclessa, Desogen, Mircette, Ortho-Cept)

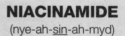

Side Effects
  Headache
  Nausea
  Postural hypotension

Nursing Considerations
  Prophylaxis and treatment
  of pellagra
  Take with meals to reduce
  GI upset, can add 325 mg
  ASA 1/2 hour before dose to
  reduce flushing
  Flushing will occur several
  hours after med taken, will
  decrease over 2 weeks
  Avoid changing positions
  (sitting/standing/lying)
  rapidly
  Rx/OTC; Preg Cat C

· ·

Side Effects
  Headache
  Dizziness
  Nausea
  Breakthrough bleeding,
  spotting

Nursing Considerations
  Prevention of pregnancy,
  treatment of endometriosis,
  hypermenorrhea (mono-
  phasic)
  Contact clinician if unusual
  bleeding, severe headache,
  difficulty breathing, changes
  in vision/coordination,
  chest/leg pain
  Avoid smoking which
  increases risk of adverse
  cardiovascular events
  Stop med for at least one
  week before surgery to
  decrease risk of thromboembolism
  Rx; Preg Cat X

ETHINYL ESTRADIOL/ETHYNODIOL
(<u>eth</u>-in-il es-tra-<u>dye</u>-ole e-thye-noe-<u>dye</u>-ole)
(Demulen)

• •

ETHINYL ESTRADIOL/ NORETHINDRONE
(<u>eth</u>-in-il es-tra-<u>dye</u>-ole nor-eth-in-drone)
(Ortho Novum 1/35)

Side Effects
Headache
Dizziness
Nausea
Breakthrough bleeding,
spotting

Nursing Considerations
Prevention of pregnancy,
treatment of endometriosis,
hypermenorrhea (mono-
phasic)
Contact clinician if unusual
bleeding, severe headache,
difficulty breathing, changes
in vision/coordination,
chest/leg pain
Avoid smoking which
increases risk of adverse
cardiovascular events
Stop med for at least one
week before surgery to
decrease risk of thrombo-
embolism
Rx; Preg Cat X

• •

Side Effects
Headache
Dizziness
Nausea
Breakthrough bleeding,
spotting

Nursing Considerations
Prevention of pregnancy,
treatment of endometriosis,
hypermenorrhea (mono-
phasic)
Contact clinician if unusual
bleeding, severe headache,
difficulty breathing, changes
in vision/coordination,
chest/leg pain
Avoid smoking which
increases risk of adverse
cardiovascular events
Stop med for at least one
week before surgery to
decrease risk of thrombo-
embolism
Rx; Preg Cat X

ETHINYL ESTRADIOL/ NORETHINDRONE
(<u>eth</u>-in-il es-tra-<u>dye</u>-ole nor-eth-<u>in</u>-drone)
(Ortho-Novum 7-7-7)

• •

ETHINYL ESTRADIOL/NORGESTREL
(<u>eth</u>-in-il es-tra-<u>dye</u>-ole nor-<u>jess</u>-trel)
(Ogestril, Ovral)

Side Effects
  Nausea

Nursing Considerations
  Female contraception
  (triphasic)
  Contact clinician if breast
  lumps, vaginal bleeding,
  edema, jaundice, dark
  urine, clay-colored stools,
  dyspnea, headache, blurred
  vision, abdominal pain,
  numbness or stiffness in
  legs, chest pain, tenderness
  with redness and swelling in
  extremities
  Contact clinician if weekly
  weight gain is over five
  pounds
  Can take with food or milk
  to decrease GI upset
  Rx; Preg Cat X

• •

Side Effects
  Headache
  Dizziness
  Nausea
  Breakthrough bleeding,
  spotting

Nursing Considerations
  Prevention of pregnancy,
  treatment of endometriosis,
  hypermenorrhea (mono-
  phasic)
  Contact clinician if unusual
  bleeding, severe headache,
  difficulty breathing, changes
  in vision/coordination,
  chest/leg pain
  Avoid smoking which
  increases risk of adverse
  cardiovascular events
  Stop med for at least one
  week before surgery to
  decrease risk of thromboembolism
  Rx; Preg Cat X

LEVONORGESTREL

(lee-voe-nor-<u>jess</u>-trel)

(Norplant, Mirena)

• •

MESTRANOL/NORETHINDRONE

(<u>mes</u>-tre-nole nor-eth-<u>in</u>-drone)

(Genora, Norinyl, Ortho-Novum)

Side Effects
Breakthrough bleeding

Nursing Considerations
Prevention of pregnancy for 5 years as a contraceptive implant; emergency contraceptive in oral form
Implant: onset 1 month, peak 1 month, duration 5 years
Implant: six capsules are implanted in the upper arm during the first 7 days after onset of menses
PO for emergency contraceptive: Given within 72 hours of unprotected intercourse and repeated 12 hours later
Rx; Preg Cat X

• •

Side Effects
Headache
Dizziness
Nausea
Breakthrough bleeding, spotting

Nursing Considerations
Prevention of pregnancy, treatment of endometriosis, hypermenorrhea (monophasic)
Contact clinician if unusual bleeding, severe headache, difficult breathing, changes in vision/coordination, chest/leg pain
Avoid smoking which increases risk of adverse cardiovascular events
Stop med for at least one week before surgery to decrease risk of thromboembolism
Rx; Preg Cat X

NORETHINDRONE
(nor-eth-<u>in</u>-drone)
(Micronor, Nor-Qd)

. . . .

NORGESTEREL
(nor-<u>jess</u>-trel)
(Ovrette)

Side Effects

Nausea

Nursing Considerations

Management of abnormal
uterine bleeding, amen-
orrhea, endometriosis,
contraception
Contact clinician if breast
lumps, vaginal bleeding,
edema, jaundice, dark
urine, clay-colored stools,
dyspnea, headache, blurred
vision, abdominal pain,
numbness or stiffness in
legs, chest pain, tenderness
with redness and swelling in
extremities
Contact clinician if weekly
weight gain is over five
pounds
Can take with food or milk
to decrease GI upset
Rx; Preg Cat X

• •

Side Effects

Nausea

Nursing Considerations

Female contraception
Contact clinician if breast
lumps, vaginal bleeding,
edema, jaundice, dark
urine, clay-colored stools,
dyspnea, headache, blurred
vision, abdominal pain,
numbness or stiffness in
legs, chest pain, tenderness
with redness and swelling in
extremities
Contact clinician if weekly
weight gain is over five
pounds
Can take with food or milk
to decrease GI upset
Rx; Preg Cat X

ESTRADIOL
(es-tra-<u>dye</u>-ole)
(Estrace)

· ·

ESTRADIOL CYPIONATE, ESTRADIOL VALERATE
(es-tra-<u>dye</u>-ole)
(Depogen, Estrasyn, Delestrogen, Valergen)

Side Effects
  Nausea
  Gynecomastia
  Testicular atrophy
  Impotence
  Contact lens intolerance

Nursing Considerations
  Oral treatment of symptoms
  of menopause, inoperable
  breast cancer (selected
  cases), prostatic cancer,
  atrophic vaginitis (cream),
  prevention of osteoporosis.
  Contact clinician if breast
  lumps, vaginal bleeding,
  edema, jaundice, dark
  urine, clay-colored stools,
  dyspnea, headache, blurred
  vision, abdominal pain,
  numbness or stiffness in
  legs, chest pain, tenderness
  with redness and swelling in
  extremities
  Men should contact clinician to report impotence or
  gynecomastia
  Contact clinician if weekly
  weight gain is over five
  pounds
  Can take with food or milk
  to decrease GI upset
  Rx; Preg Cat X

• •

Side Effects
  Contact lens intolerance
  Gynecomastia
  Testicular atrophy
  Impotence

Nursing Considerations
  Treatment of symptoms
  of menopause, inoperable
  breast cancer (selected
  cases), prostatic cancer,
  atrophic vaginitis, prevention of osteoporosis
  Contact clinician if breast
  lumps, vaginal bleeding,
  edema, jaundice, dark
  urine, clay-colored stools,
  dyspnea, headache, blurred
  vision, abdominal pain,
  numbness or stiffness in
  legs, chest pain, tenderness
  with redness and swelling in
  extremities
  Men should contact clinician to report impotence or
  gynecomastia
  Contact clinician if weekly
  weight gain is over five
  pounds
  Give IM injection deeply in
  large muscle mass
  Rx; Preg Cat X

ESTRADIOL PATCH
(es-tra-<u>dye</u>-ole)
(Alora, Climara, Esclim, Estraderm, Fempatch)

• •

MEDROXYPROGESTRONE ACETATE
(me-drox-ee-proe-<u>jess</u>-te-rone)
(Provera, Depo-Provera)

Side Effects
Contact lens intolerance
Gynecomastia
Testicular atrophy
Impotence

Nursing Considerations
Treatment of symptoms of menopause, inoperable breast cancer (selected cases), prostatic cancer, atrophic vaginitis, prevention of osteoporosis
Contact clinician if breast lumps, vaginal bleeding, edema, jaundice, dark urine, clay-colored stools, dyspnea, headache, blurred vision, abdominal pain, numbness or stiffness in legs, chest pain, tenderness with redness and swelling in extremities
Men should contact clinician to report impotence or gynecomastia
Contact clinician if weekly weight gain is over five pounds
Apply patch to trunk of body twice a week; press firmly and hold in place for 10 seconds to ensure good contact
Rx; Preg Cat X

• •

Side Effects
Nausea
Testicular atrophy
Impotence
Contact lens intolerance

Nursing Considerations
Management of abnormal uterine bleeding, secondary amenorrhea, endometrial cancer, renal cancer, contraceptive, prevent endometrial changes associated with estrogen replacement therapy
Contact clinician if weekly weight gain is over five pounds
Give IM injection deeply in large muscle mass, rotate sites, injection may be painful
Use with caution with history of depression
Contact clinician if swelling in calves, sudden chest pain or shortness of breath
(Rx; Preg Cat D)

Joint Commission on Accreditation of Healthcare List of "Do Not Use" Abbreviations

One hundred percent compliance, in all forms of clinical documentation, with a reasonably comprehensive list of prohibited "dangerous" abbreviations, acronyms and symbols continues to be the long-term objective of the Joint Commission. The following items must be included on each accredited organization's "Do not use" list as of May 2005:

Abbreviation	Potential Problem	Preferred Term
U (for unit)	Mistaken for "0" (zero), the number "4" (four), or "cc."	Write "unit"
IU (for International Unit)	Mistaken for "IV" (intravenous) or the number "10" (ten).	Write "International Unit"
Q.D., QD, q.d., qd (daily) Q.O.D., QOD, q.o.d., qod (every other day)	Mistaken for each other. The period after the Q can be mistaken for an "I" and the "O" can be mistaken for "I"	Write "daily" and "every other day"
Trailing zero (X.0 mg), Lack of leading zero (.X mg)	Decimal point is missed	Write X mg Write 0.X mg
MS MSO$_4$ MgSO$_4$	Confused for one another. Can mean morphine sulfate or magnesium sulfate.	Write "morphine sulfate" Write "magnesium sulfate"

In addition to the "minimum required list" above, the following items should also be considered for organizational "do not use" lists. These all may possibly be included in future "Do Not Use" list.

Abbreviation	Potential Problem	Preferred Term
> (greater than) < (less than)	Misinterpreted as the number "7" (seven) or the letter "L" Confused for one another	Write "greater than" Write "less than"
Abbreviations for drug names	Misinterpreted due to similar abbreviations for multiple drugs	Write drug names in full
Apothecary units	Unfamiliar to many practitioners Confused with metric units	Use metric units
@	Mistaken for the number "2" (two)	Write "at"
cc	Mistaken for U (units) when poorly written	Write "ml" or "milliliters"
µg	Mistaken for mg (milligrams) resulting in one thousand-fold overdose	Write "mcg" or "micrograms"

Note: An abbreviation on the "do not use" list should not be used in any of its forms—upper or lower case; with or without periods.

The Institute for Safe Medication Practices (ISMP) has published a list of dangerous abbreviations relating to medication use that it recommends should be explicitly prohibited. This list is available on the ISMP website: *www.ismp.org*.

Source: Joint Commission on Accreditation of Heathcare Organizations, *www.jcaho.org*. Reprinted with permission.

Appendix B: Controlled Substance Schedules

Drugs regulated by the Controlled Substances Act of 1970 are classified:

Schedule I: High abuse potential and no accepted medical use. Examples include heroin, marijuana, and LSD.

Schedule II: High abuse potential with severe dependence liability. Examples include narcotics, amphetamines, and some barbiturates.

Schedule III: Less abuse potential than schedule II drugs and moderate dependence liability. Examples include nonbarbiturate sedatives, nonamphetamine stimulants, anabolic steroids, and limited amounts of certain narcotics.

Schedule IV: Less abuse potential than schedule III drugs and limited dependence liability. Examples include some sedatives, anxiolytics, and nonnarcotic analgesics.

Schedule V: Limited abuse potential. Examples include small amounts of narcotics, such as codeine, used as antidiarrheals or antitussives.

Appendix C: Pregnancy Risk Categories

The FDA has assigned the following pregnancy risk categories:

Category A: Adequate studies in pregnant women have failed to show a risk to the fetus in the first trimester (and there is not evidence of risk in later trimesters) and the possibility of fetal harm appears remote.

Category B: Animal studies haven't shown a risk to the fetus, but controlled studies haven't been conducted in pregnant women; or animal studies have shown an adverse effect on the fetus, but adequate studies in pregnant women haven't shown a risk to the fetus.

Category C: Animal studies have shown an adverse effect on the fetus, but adequate studies haven't been conducted in pregnant women. The benefits may be acceptable despite the risks.

Category D: The drug may cause a risk to the fetus, but potential benefits may be acceptable despite the risks (life-threatening situation or serious disease).

Category X: Animal or human studies show fetal abnormalities, or adverse reaction reports indicate evidence of fetal risk. The risks involved clearly outweigh potential benefits.

NA: Rating is not available

APPENDIX D: COMMON MEDICAL ABBREVIATIONS

ABC—airway, breathing, circulation

abd.—abdomen

ABG—arterial blood gas

ABO—system of classifying blood groups

ac—before meals

ACE—angiotensin converting enzyme

ACS—acute compartment syndrome

ACTH—adrenocorticotrophic hormone

ADH—antidiuretic hormone

ADL—activities of daily living

ad lib—freely, as desired

AFP—alpha-fetoprotein

AIDS—acquired immunodeficiency syndrome

AKA—above the knee amputation

ALL—acute lymphocytic leukemia

ALS—amyotrophic lateral sclerosis

ALT—alkaline phosphatase (formerly SGPT)

AMI—antibody-mediated immunity

AML—acute myelogenous leukemia

amt.—amount

ANA—antinuclear antibody

ANS—autonomic nervous system

AP—anteroposterior

A&P—anterior and posterior

APC—atrial premature contraction

aq.—water

ARDS—adult respiratory distress syndrome

ASD—atrial septal defect

ASHD—atherosclerotic heart disease

AST—aspartate aminotransferase (formerly SGOT)

ATP—adenosine triphosphate

AV—atrioventricular

BCG—Bacille Calmette-Guerin

bid—two times a day

BKA—below the knee amputation

BLS—basic life support

BMR—basal metabolic rate

BP—blood pressure

BPH—benign prostatic hypertrophy

bpm—beats per minute

BPR—bathroom privileges

BSA—body surface area

BUN—blood, urea, nitrogen

C—centigrade, Celsius

c̄—with

Ca—calcium

CA—cancer

CABG—coronary artery bypass graft

CAD—coronary artery disease

CAPD—continuous ambulatory peritoneal dialysis

caps—capsules

CBC—complete blood count

CC—chief complaint

CCU—coronary care unit, critical care unit

CDC—Centers for Disease Control and Prevention

CHF—congestive heart failure

CK—creatine kinase

Cl—chloride

CLL—chronic lymphocytic leukemia

cm—centimeter

CMV—cytomegalovirus infection

CNS—central nervous system

CO—carbon monoxide, cardiac output

CO_2—carbon dioxide

comp—compound

cont—continuous

COPD—chronic obstructive pulmonary disease

CP—cerebral palsy

CPAP—continuous positive airway pressure

CPK—creatine phosphokinase

CPR—cardiopulmonary resuscitation

CRP—C-reactive protein

C&S—culture and sensitivity

CSF—cerebrospinal fluid

CT—computerized tomography

CTD—connective tissue disease

CTS—carpal tunnel syndrome

cu—cubic

CVA—cerebrovascular accident or costovertebral angle

CVC—central venous catheter

CVP—central venous pressure

DC—discontinue

D&C—dilation and curettage

DIC—disseminated intravascular coagulation

DIFF—differential blood count

dil.—dilute

DJD—degenerative joint disease

DKA—diabetic ketoacidosis

dL—deciliter (100 ml)

DM—diabetes mellitus

DNA—deoxyribonucleic acid

DNR—do not resuscitate

DO—doctor of osteopathy

DOE—dyspnea on exertion

DPT—vaccine for diphtheria, pertussis, tetanus

Dr.—doctor

DVT—deep vein thrombosis

D/W—dextrose in water

Dx—diagnosis

ECF—extracellular fluid

ECG or EKG—electrocardiogram

ECT—electroconvulsive therapy

ED—emergency department

EEG—electroencephalogram

EMD—electromechanical dissociation

EMG—electromyography
ENT—ear, nose, and throat
ESR—erythrocyte sedimentation rate
ESRD—end stage renal disease
ET—endotracheal tube
F—Fahrenheit
FBD—fibrocystic breast disease
FBS—fasting blood sugar
FDA—Food and Drug Administration
FFP—fresh frozen plasma
fl—fluid
4 • 4—piece of gauze 4" by 4" used for dressings
FSH—follicle-stimulating hormone
ft.—foot, feet (unit of measure)
FUO—fever of undetermined origin
g, gm—gram
GB—gall bladder
GFR—glomerular filtration rate
GH—growth hormone
GI—gastrointestinal
gr—grain
GSC—Glasgow coma scale
gtts—drops
GU—genitourinary
GYN—gynecological
h or hrs—hour or hours
(H)—hypodermically
Hb or Hgb—hemoglobin
HCG—human chorionic gonadotropin
HCO_3^-—bicarbonate
Hct—hematocrit

HD—hemodialysis
HDL—high-density lipoproteins
Hg—mercury
Hgb—hemoglobin
HGH—human growth hormone
HHNC—hyperglycemia hyperosmolar nonketotic coma
HIV—human immunodeficiency virus
HLA—human leukocyte antigen
HR—heart rate
hr—hour
HSV—herpes simplex virus
HTN—hypertension
H_2O—water
Hx—history
Hz—hertz (cycles/second)
IABP—intra-aortic balloon pump
IBBP—intermittent positive pressure breathing
IBS—irritable bowel syndrome
ICF—intracellular fluid
ICP—increased intracranial pressure
ICS—intercostal space
ICU—intensive care unit
IDDM—insulin dependent diabetes mellitus
IgA—immunoglobulin A
IM—intramuscular
I&O—intake and output
IOP—increased intraocular pressure
IPG—impedance plethysmogram

IPPB—intermittent positive-pressure breathing
IUD—intrauterine device
IV—intravenous
IVC—intraventricular catheter
IVP—intravenous pyelogram
JRA—juvenile rheumatoid arthritis
K⁺—potassium
kcal—kilocalorie (food calorie)
kg—kilogram
KO, KVO—keep vein open
KS—Kaposi's sarcoma
KUB—kidneys, ureters, bladder
L, l—liter
lab—laboratory
lb.—pound
LBBB—left bundle branch block
LDH—lactate dehydrogenase
LDL—low-density lipoproteins
LE—lupus erythematosus
LH—luteinizing hormone
liq—liquid
LLQ—left lower quadrant
LOC—level of consciousness
LP—lumbar puncture
LPN, LVN—licensed practical or vocational nurse
Lt, lt—left
LTC—long term care
LUQ—left upper quadrant
LV—left ventricle
m—minum, meter, micron
MAO—monoamine oxidase inhibitors

MAST—military antishock trousers
mcg—microgram
MCH—mean corpuscular hemoglobin
MCV—mean corpuscular volume
MD—muscular dystrophy, medical doctor
MDI—metered dose inhaler
mEq—milliequivalent
mg—milligram
Mg—magnesium
MG—myasthenia gravis
MI—myocardial infarction
ml—milliliter
mm—millimeter
MMR—vaccine for measles, mumps, rubella
MRI—magnetic resonance imaging
MS—multiple sclerosis
N—nitrogen, normal (strength of solution)
NIDDM—non-insulin dependent diabetes mellitus
Na⁺—sodium
NaCl—sodium chloride
NANDA—North American Nursing Diagnosis Association
NG—nasogastric
NGT—nasogastric tube
NLN—National League for Nursing
noc—at night
NPO—nothing by mouth
NS—normal saline
NSAIDS—nonsteroidal anti-inflammatory

drugs

NSNA—National Student Nurses' Association

NST—non-stress test

O₂—oxygen

OB-GYN—obstetrics and gynecology

OCT—oxytocin challenge test

OOB—out of bed

OPC—outpatient clinic

OR—operating room

o̅s—by mouth

OSHA—Occupational Safety and Health Administration

OTC—over the counter (drug that can be obtained without a prescription)

oz.—ounce

p̅—with

P—pulse, pressure, phosphorus

PA Chest—posterior-anterior chest x-ray

PAC—premature atrial complexes

PaCO₂—partial pressure of carbon dioxide in arterial blood

PaO₂—partial pressure of oxygen in arterial blood

PAD—peripheral artery disease

Pap—Papanicolaou smear

pc—after meals

PCA—patient controlled analgesia

PCO₂—partial pressure of carbon dioxide

PCP—Pneumocystis carinii pneumonia

PD—peritoneal dialysis

PE—pulmonary embolism

PEEP—positive end-expiratory pressure

PERRLA—pupils equal, round, react to light and accommodation

PET—postural emission tomography

PFT—pulmonary function tests

pH—hydrogen ion concentration

PID—pelvic inflammatory disease

PKD—polycystic disease

PKU—phenylketonuria

PMS—premenstrual syndrome

PND—paroxysmal nocturnal dyspnea

PO, po—by mouth

PO₂—partial pressure of oxygen

PPD—positive purified protein derivative (of tuberculin)

PPN—partial parenteral nutrition

PRN, prn—as needed, whenever necessary

pro time—prothrombin time

PSA—prostate-specific antigen

psi—pounds per square inch

PSP—phenol-sulfonphthalein

PT—physical therapy, prothrombin time

PTCA—percutaneous transluminal coronary angioplasty

PTH—parathyroid hormone
PTT—partial thromboplastin time
PUD—peptic ulcer disease
PVC—premature ventricular contraction
q—every
QA—quality assurance
qh—every hour
q 2 h—every two hours
q 4 h—every four hours
qid—four times a day
qs—quantity sufficient
R—rectal temperature, respirations, roentgen
RA—rheumatoid arthritis
RAI—radioactive iodine
RAIU—radioactive iodine uptake
RAS—reticular activating system
RBBB—right bundle branch block
RBC—red blood cell or count
RCA—right coronary artery
RDA—recommended dietary allowance
resp—respirations
RF—rheumatic fever, rheumatoid factor
Rh—antigen on blood cell indicated by + or –
RIND—reversible ischemic neurologic deficit
RLQ—right lower quadrant
RN—registered nurse
RNA—ribonucleic acid
R/O, r/o—rule out, to exclude
ROM—range of motion (of joint)
Rt, rt—right

RUQ—right upper quadrant
Rx—prescription
$\bar{s}$—without
S. or Sig.—(Signa) to write on label
SA—sinoatrial node
SaO_2—systemic arterial oxygen saturation (%)
sat sol—saturated solution
SBE—subacute bacterial endocarditis
SDA—same day admission
SDS—same day surgery
sed rate—sedimentation rate
SGOT—serum glutamic-oxaloacetic transaminase (see AST)
SGPT—serum glutamic-pyruvic transaminase (see ALT)
SI—International System of Units
SIADH—syndrome of inappropriate antidiuretic hormone
SIDS—sudden infant death syndrome
SL—sublingual
SLE—systemic lupus erythematosus
SOB—short of breath
sol—solution
SMBG—self-monitoring blood glucose
SMR—submucous resection
sp gr—specific gravity
spec.—specimen
$\overline{ss}$—one half
SS—soap suds
SSKI—saturated solution of potassium iodide

stat—immediately
STD—sexually transmitted disease
subcut—subcutaneous
sx—symptoms
Syr.—syrup
T—temperature, thoracic to be followed by the number designating specific thoracic vertebra
T&A—tonsillectomy and adenoidectomy
tabs—tablets
TB—tuberculosis
T&C—type and crossmatch
TED—antiembolitic stockings
temp—temperature
TENS—transcutaneous electrical nerve stimulation
TIA—transient ischemic attack
TIBC—total iron binding capacity
tid—three times a day
tinct, or tr.—tincture
TMJ—temporomandibular joint
t-pa, TPA—tissue plasminogen activator
TPN—total parenteral nutrition
TPR—temperature, pulse, respiration
TQM—total quality management
TSE—testicular self-examination
TSH—thyroid-stimulating hormone

tsp—teaspoon
TSS—toxic shock syndrome
TURP—transuretheral prostatectomy
UA—urinalysis
ung—ointment
URI—upper respiratory tract infection
UTI—urinary tract infection
VAD—venous access device
VDRL—Veneral Disease Research laboratory (test for syphilis)
VF, Vfib—ventricular fibrillation
VPC—ventricular premature complexes
VS, vs—vital signs
VSD—ventricular septal defect
VT—ventricular tachycardia
WBC—white blood cell or count
WHO—World Health Organization
wt—weight

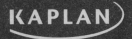